MENTAL HEALTH SERVICES
FOR THE MENTALLY RETARDED

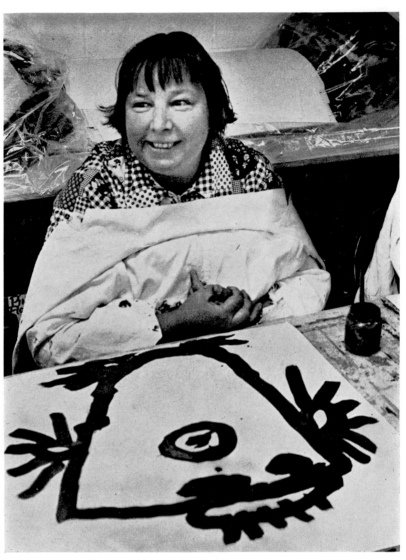

"I did it!"
(*Photo by Richard Berger*)

Mental Health Services for the Mentally Retarded

Edited by

ELIAS KATZ, Ph.D.

Assistant Director
Center for Training in Community Psychiatry
and Mental Health Administration
Berkeley, California

Lecturer in Psychology
Department of Psychiatry
School of Medicine
University of California
San Francisco, California

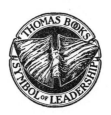

CHARLES C THOMAS · PUBLISHER
Springfield · Illinois · U.S.A.

Published and Distributed Throughout the World by

CHARLES C THOMAS • PUBLISHER

BANNERSTONE HOUSE

301-327 East Lawrence Avenue, Springfield, Illinois, U.S.A.

© 1972, by CHARLES C THOMAS • PUBLISHER

ISBN 0-398-02516-9

Library of Congress Catalog Card Number: 74-190327

Printed in the United States of America

C-24

CONTRIBUTORS

Virginia Y. Blacklidge, M.D., M.P.H.

Chief of Service
Alameda County Mental Retardation
    Service
Oakland, California

Peter Cohen, M.D.

Associate Professor
Department of Pediatrics
University of California
San Francisco, California

Leon Cytryn, M.D.

Research Associate
Children's Hospital of the D.C.
Associate Professor of Pediatric
    Psychiatry
George Washington University
    School of Medicine
Washington, D.C.

Sheldon R. Gelman, A.C.S.W.

Assistant Professor of Sociology
Pennsylvania State University
University Park, Pennsylvania

Portia Bell Hume, M.D.

Clinical Professor of Psychiatry,
    Emeritus
School of Medicine
University of California
San Francisco, California

Elias Katz, Ph.D.

Assistant Director
Center for Training in Community

Psychiatry and Mental Health
    Administration
Department of Mental Hygiene
Berkeley, California
Lecturer in Psychology
Department of Psychiatry
School of Medicine
University of California
San Francisco, California

Henry Leland, Ph.D.

Chief Psychologist
Herschel C. Nisonger Center for
    Mental Retardation
Associate Professor of Psychology
Ohio State University
Columbus, Ohio

Leopold Lippman

Director of Services for the Mentally
    and Physically Handicapped
City of New York
New York, New York

Reginald S. Lourie, M.D.

Director
Department of Psychiatry
Children's Hospital of the D.C.
Medical Director
Hillcrest Children's Center
Professor of Psychiatry
The George Washington University
    School of Medicine
Washington, D.C.

Florence Ludins-Katz, M.A.

Art Consultant
Berkeley, California

Frank J. Menolascino, M.D.

Clinical Director
Division of Preventive and Social
*   Psychiatry*
Nebraska Psychiatric Institute
College of Medicine
University of Nebraska
Omaha, Nebraska

Stanley Meyers

Northeast Regional Representative
National Association for Retarded
*   Children*
New York, New York

Nathan B. Miron, Ph.D.

Senior Psychologist
Sonoma State Hospital
Eldridge, California
Staff Psychologist
Behavior Therapy Institute
Sausalito, California

Charles M. Moody, M.S.W.

Chief, Mental Retardation Services
San Joaquin Mental Health Services
Stockton, California

Ernest F. Pecci, M.D.

Medical Chief of the Multipurpose
*   Centers*
Chief, Child Development Clinic
Contra Costa County Mental Health
*   Services*
Martinez, California

Arthur Segal, A.C.S.W.

Mental Health Coordinator
Health Services Division
Marin County Community Mental
*   Health Services*
San Rafael, California

Irwin M. Shapiro, M.D.

Associate Director
Center for Training in Community
*   Psychiatry and Mental Health*
*   Administration*
Department of Mental Hygiene
Berkeley, California
Assistant Clinical Professor of
*   Psychiatry*
School of Medicine
University of California
San Francisco, California

R. K. Janmeja Singh, Ph.D.

Lecturer
California School of Professional
*   Psychology*
San Francisco, California
Assistant Director
Center for Training in Community
*   Psychiatry and Mental Health*
*   Administration*
Berkeley, California

Daniel E. Smith, Ph.D.

Psychologist
Parsons State Hospital and
*   Training Center*
Parsons, Kansas

Irving R. Stone, M.A.

Assistant for Hospital-Community
*   Programming*
Fairview State Hospital
Costa Mesa, California

To Florence

PREFACE

THE purpose of this book is to throw light on a subject which is of growing concern to those who work with the mentally retarded and their families—mental health services for the mentally retarded.

This book has developed out of the belief that many of the mentally retarded suffer from acute and chronic emotional disturbances and behavior disorders and that there is relatively little provision for mental health services to help them. Each contributor in his own way has identified in what ways the mentally retarded are a population at risk of mental breakdown, and has indicated directions which can be followed to prevent such breakdowns and to provide appropriate help for those who urgently need it.

Although its coverage is broad, this book makes no pretense of being exhaustive. The varied professional backgrounds of the contributors and their individual writing styles reflect the breadth of concern. The many-faceted aspects of this problem must call into play many different approaches.

ELIAS KATZ

NOTE: The contents of this book are the responsibility of the authors and do not necessarily reflect the policies and procedures of the California Department of Mental Hygiene or of the Center for Training in Community Psychiatry and Mental Health Administration at Berkeley.

ACKNOWLEDGMENTS

IT is a pleasure to acknowledge the contributors to this book. Their willingness to share thinking and experience in a relatively uncharted area has not only made my editorial task stimulating and rewarding, but should encourage discussion and soul-searching among our many co-workers in the field.

I am grateful to my colleagues on the staff of the Center for Training in Community Psychiatry and Mental Health Administration at Berkeley,* Donald T. Brown, M.D., Portia Bell Hume, M.D., Irwin M. Shapiro, M.D., and R. K. Janmeja Singh, Ph.D., for stimulating interactions contributing much to my thinking as to the relationships between mental health and mental retardation. To Dr. Hume I owe not only a greater awareness of the theoretical framework underlying this book, but constructive support in developing the training program in mental retardation described in Chapter 18. I also thank the faculty of the Center, some of whose lectures found their way into this volume.

A special debt of gratitude is owed to the students from many agencies and many disciplines who have participated in the mental retardation training program at the Center. They and their co-workers have provided the necessary interaction which has done much to shape thinking and practice in this field.

Above all, I wish to acknowledge the part played by the mentally retarded and their parents and caretakers. Their need for help in dealing with incredibly difficult problems have left indelible imprints on the feelings and actions of professionals, and have motivated this book's efforts to improve delivery of mental health services for the mentally retarded.

ELIAS KATZ

---

* A postgraduate training facility of the California State Department of Mental Hygiene.

CONTENTS

MENTAL HEALTH SERVICES
FOR THE MENTALLY RETARDED

Chapter 1

INTRODUCTION

W HO are the mentally retarded? What are their needs for mental health services? What mental health services are currently being provided? What directions should be pursued to provide mental health services for the mentally retarded?

WHO ARE THE MENTALLY RETARDED

Most professionals in the fields of mental health and mental retardation in the United States are likely to use as their frame of reference the *American Journal of Mental Deficiency* definition[1,2] which has been adopted by the American Psychiatric Association:[3]

"Mental retardation refers to subaverage general intellectual functioning which originates during the development period and is associated with impairment in adaptive behavior."

Let us review briefly the mental health implications of this definition.

The term "subaverage general intellectual functioning" conceptualizes intelligence (general intellectual functioning) as a measurable human trait expressed as an IQ score which is distributed along a continuum, in a "normal" distribution around a midpoint known as the average or mean, 100 IQ. Those with the highest IQ scores are considered the "gifted" intellectually, and those with lowest IQ scores are the "mentally retarded."

An important property of the "normal" curve is that the theoretical distribution of IQ scores in the population can be predicted statistically. Thus, about 16 per cent of the total population falls below one standard deviation from the mean, and about 3 per cent of the total population falls below two standard deviations from the mean. If one assumes that one standard devia-

3

tion is equivalent to 15 IQ points, this would suggest that about 16 per cent (32,000,000 persons out of a population of 200,000,000) have IQ scores below 85, and about 3 per cent (6,000,000 persons out of a population of 200,000,000) have IQ scores below 70.

In the *American Journal of Mental Deficiency* definition, "subaverage general intellectual functioning" refers to all those who fall below one standard deviation from the mean, below 85 IQ.

The size of the mentally retarded population at risk of mental breakdown has important theoretical and practical implications for the delivery of mental health services. If we use the lower figure of 3 per cent of the population as being mentally retarded, the needs for mental health services for 6,000,000 people are staggering, but if we use the higher figure of 16 per cent, the sheer volume of needed services is overwhelming.

The phrase "originates during the developmental period" strongly reinforces the concept that mental retardation is an integral component of each individual's growth and development from the moment of conception until growth has ceased. Such a concept is applicable not only to physical development but to emotional and social development. It has many implications for intervention and treatment of the mental disorders of childhood and adolescence which may adversely affect an individual's "general intellectual functioning." It also has many implications for changing the social environment for the developing child so that destructive emotional trauma can be reduced or eliminated.

The phrase "associated with impairment in adaptive behavior" has much to offer relative to mental health services. From a theoretical viewpoint, "adaptive behavior" may be conceptualized as being distributed like other human traits ("intelligence," "height," "weight," etc.) in a "normal" curve around a hypothetical average or mean. Perhaps the most important mental health implication of this portion of the definition is that adaptive behavior can be modified. It may not be possible to substantially improve the mentally retarded individual's intellectual ability. However, it has been amply demonstrated that his behavior in adjusting to his environment can be substantially improved through learning appropriate skills and knowledges, and through developing an improved self-image.

WHAT ARE THEIR NEEDS FOR MENTAL
HEALTH SERVICES?

The needs of the mentally retarded can be viewed in two ways, in terms of basic physiological and psychosocial needs of all human beings, and in terms of the needs of the retarded for mental health services to alleviate their emotional disorders.

Human needs whether for the normal or mentally retarded may be broadly classified as physiological and psychosocial, although these needs are often interdependent and overlapping. Physiological needs include the need for food, clothing, and shelter in order to survive, and the need to reproduce the species. Psychosocial needs encompass needs for security, which arise from needs for companionship and love as well as needs to acquire possessions and property, and needs for adequacy, which in turn arise from needs to achieve status and prestige, needs to control others, and needs to be independent.

Failure to satisfy basic needs often leads to impairment in adaptive behavior. Among the mentally retarded in addition to the usual obstacles which stand in the way of meeting needs, other obstacles are often added: a long history of failure in competition with normal and bright associates, general slowness in learning, poor communication skills, social and cultural deprivation. These factors may eventuate in serious forms of mental disorder, including neurotic or psychotic reactions. The whole gamut of mental illness has been identified among the mentally retarded.

Help for the emotionally disturbed mentally retarded depends on such factors as the nature of the mental illness and associated maladaptive behavior, the degree to which disturbed behavior affects others around him, and the availability of trained staff and facilities to handle the disturbed person. The fact that so many retarded individuals have trouble in thinking conceptually and in expressing their ideas in itself creates serious frustration and strengthens feelings of inadequacy and worthlessness. Many have learned to suppress their fears or antagonism through an outward show of docility and conformity, which sometimes erupts in self-destructive or homicidal acts. Still others have tested the limits of tolerance for their abnormal behavior among their teachers, parents, or neighbors, and have learned how far they can go without being forcibly restrained or removed from the situation.

WHAT ARE THE MENTAL HEALTH SERVICES FOR THE MENTALLY RETARDED?

There are several ways in which mental health services for the mentally retarded can be classified. For present purposes, such services will be grouped as "direct services" and "indirect" (or "supportive")[4] services. Such classifications are of course quite arbitrary, since in practice they often overlap.

"Direct" services include early case finding and evaluation, crisis intervention, individual counseling and psychotherapy, group psychotherapy, behavior modification, and other treatment modalities, including the use of drugs. "Indirect" or "supportive" services include manpower development and utilization, research, mental health consultation, and community organization of services.

WHAT MENTAL HEALTH SERVICES ARE CURRENTLY BEING PROVIDED?

It is impossible to determine what direct or indirect mental health services are being provided on behalf of the mentally retarded. Some seriously emotionally disturbed retarded children and adults are being provided with direct mental health services, whether by private practitioners, in mental health clinics, or in mental hospitals. It is likely that those who do receive this type of help are only a small fraction of those in distress who need direct services.

Numerous studies have indicated that use of available health services (including mental health services) varies directly with income, the poor using them the least. Other studies have indicated that the prevalence of mental disorder is related to socioeconomic class, with higher prevalence in the lower classes. Still other studies have indicated that there is a far greater number of mentally retarded, especially the moderately and mildly retarded in the lower socioeconomic classes.[8] Putting these findings together, it would appear that emotionally disturbed mentally retarded individuals in the lower socioeconomic classes probably make little use of available mental health services.

Not only has there been relatively limited use of direct mental health services, such as individual and group psychotherapy with the mentally retarded, but little use has been made of an important form of indirect mental health services: mental health consultation. In a few communities mental health consultation is provided for teachers of special classes for mentally retarded children and for staffs of sheltered workshops serving mentally retarded adults. The aim is to assist workers in dealing with the mental health problems of the retarded in the classroom or work situation.

WHAT DIRECTIONS SHOULD BE PURSUED TO PROVIDE MENTAL HEALTH SERVICES FOR THE MENTALLY RETARDED?

Principles underlying the delivery of mental health services for the mentally retarded must be based on a broad faith in the dignity of man, and a strong belief in social responsibility for enabling all men to enjoy inalienable rights of security and freedom.[5, 6] The following principles reflect current thinking in this area:

1. Wherever possible, the retarded should be integrated into normal community living (Normalization Principle).

2. Every effort should be made to expand the retardate's capabilities to replace disruptive behavior patterns with socially appropriate ways of interacting.

3. Mental health services should be available to mentally retarded in the same amount and quality as they are available to all other citizens in the community.

4. A comprehensive continuum of mental health services should be available and accessible to every retarded person.

5. Coordination must exist among public and private agencies, and individuals providing mental health services to the mentally retarded.

6. A fixed point of referral and information in the commu-

nity should be available, with opportunity for life-time consultation and referral to which every retarded person and his family could turn for guidance and help as needed.

7. All sectors of the community should be involved in the planning, implementation, and evaluation of mental health services for the mentally retarded.

Every effort must be made to deliver basic health services (including mental health services) to all persons who need them. It is most unfortunate that large segments in our society (encompassing those of low-income and/or in minority groups among whom are found many mentally retarded persons) are not being provided with needed health services, even though they are eligible for them. Our first responsibility is to insure that needed services are provided for all.

We must seek to reduce and eventually eliminate the stereotypes which have developed in the thinking and practice of many mental health professionals that no mentally retarded person can profit from mental health services such as counseling and psychotherapy. It is true that severely and profoundly retarded persons may not be benefitted by traditional psychotherapeutic methods. However, they constitute only a small fraction of the retarded population. The vast proportion of the mildly and moderately retarded can and do respond as well as normal persons to mental health services.

It must be kept in mind that emotionally disturbed mentally retarded persons are essentially powerless to act for themselves. This means that they need strong advocates to support mental health services on their behalf. Mental health professionals who believe that the retarded should be provided with needed mental health services must join with parents, community leaders, legislators, and other professionals in demanding improved services, staff, and facilities.

One approach to improving the delivery of mental health services for the mentally retarded is to bring together current theory and practice. The previously unpublished papers in this volume are intended to provide a picture of the "state of the art" at present, and to give stimulus as to future directions.

Portia Bell Hume's article provides a theoretical framework

from her wealth of experience in community psychiatry. The papers by R. K. Janmeja Singh, Henry Leland and Daniel E. Smith, Charles M. Moody, Frank J. Menolascino, Nathan B. Miron, Sheldon R. Gelman, and Florence Ludins-Katz are concerned with direct mental health services, whether in terms of psychotherapy, behavior modification, creative art expression, or institutional programming. Ernest Pecci highlights the importance of working with parents and siblings of the retarded, since the whole family is so often involved, while Peter Cohen gives an indication of the physician's role in dealing with the child, the family, and community resources. Irwin M. Shapiro, Leon Cytryn and Reginald S. Lourie provide an understanding of basic approaches to prevention of mental illness in the mentally retarded. Virginia Y. Blacklidge gives some pointers on handling of sexual adjustment problems. Irving Stone, Leopold Lippman and Stanley E. Meyer, and Arthur Segal develop insights into the mental retardation service delivery system, as seen from the viewpoint of the institution, the community and the individual. The concluding paper by the writer describes a training program for practitioners who provide mental health services for the mentally retarded.

Rather than attempt to extract generalizations from these papers, it may be more useful to point to the generally optimistic and favorable feeling tone expressed towards the mentally retarded by each contributor. While recognizing that the mentally retarded have handicaps of greater or less severity, nevertheless each writer in his own way expresses belief that the mentally retarded can be helped, and draws upon experience to demonstrate the validity of his faith. That leaders in this field can approach their task in these terms provides our greatest hope for the best and most effective delivery of mental health services to the mentally retarded.

REFERENCES

1. Heber, Rick (Ed.): A manual on terminology and classification in mental retardation. Monograph supplement. *Am J Ment Defic,* 64(2):3, 1958.
2. Heber, Rick: Modifications in the manual on terminology and classification in mental retardation. *Am J Ment Defic,* 65:499, 1961.
3. American Psychiatric Association: *Diagnostic and Statistical Manual*

   of Mental Disorders, 2nd Edition (DSM-II). Washington, D.C., Author, 1968.
4. Gardner, William I. and Nisonger, Herschel W.: A manual on program development in mental retardation. Monograph supplement. *Am J Ment Defic,* 66(4), 1962.
5. Katz, Elias: *The Retarded Adult in the Community*. Springfield, Ill., Charles C Thomas, 1968.
6. Katz, Elias: The *Retarded Adult at Home: A Guide for Parents*. Seattle, Wash., Special Child Publications, Inc., 1970.
7. Menolascino, Frank J. (Ed.): *Psychiatric Approaches to Mental Retardation*. New York, Basic Books, Inc., 1970.
8. President's Committee on Mental Retardation: *MR 70, The Decisive Decade*. Washington, D.C., U.S. Government Printing Office, 1971.

Chapter 2

DIRECT AND INDIRECT MENTAL HEALTH SERVICES FOR THE MENTALLY RETARDED

INTRODUCTION

IN community mental health practice today, it is recognized that within the total population at risk of mental breakdown there are individuals who are at special risk because of deficits. There are two main sources of such handicaps. On the one hand, deficits occur in the form of personal deficiencies that limit an individual's inherent capacity to develop in accordance with the average expectable timetable, and to cope with the external world as effectively as the average person. On the other hand, a shortage of necessary supplies from the external world may halt or slow down the developmental processes through which every member of the human species learns to cope with the average, expectable environment. Those who are recognized, presumably correctly, as mentally retarded suffer from both kinds of deficits. Furthermore, their needs are greater than the average person's and the responses of the external world may be too little or too late.

Mental health services for the mentally retarded include more than direct, remedial measures of psychiatric, neurological, and general medical or pediatric kinds that focus on an illness diagnosed as some form of mental retardation. Rather, the emphasis upon the mental health of the retarded implies not only that the handicap of mental retardation may be reduced, if not eliminated, through preventive types of intervention, but also that mental retardation does not confer immunity on its victims to many of the same kinds of mental breakdown that occur in the rest of the population. The presence of mental retardation enhances the risk of mental breakdown, to be sure, as do other severe handicaps. Furthermore, a mentally retarded person may easily acquire secondary handicaps of a physical, psychosocial, educational, or occupational nature, for example. Consequently, the mentally retarded need mental health services at least as much as, or more than, those who are not so manifestly encumbered. A realistic appraisal of the degree and precise nature of the handicap in the mentally retarded is clearly essential; what may not be so obvious is that both the care-taking and the care-giving systems needed by the mentally retarded are hampered by widely held and generally unquestioned stereotypes, or by personal attitudes that interfere with the delivery of habilitative, educational, and rehabilitative services of various kinds.

PREVENTION

Preventive interventions in behalf of the mentally retarded need not be confined to eugenics and the elimination of congenital casualties, brain-damaging illnesses, or head injuries, important as all such efforts certainly are. On the contrary, postnatal deprivations plus predictable, developmental and unpredictable, accidental life-crises may either worsen the inborn forms of mental retardation or be wholly responsible for the secondary or acquired characteristics of arrest, regression, or slowing down of mental development. Primary prevention aimed at the reduction in the number of new cases must, therefore, be addressed not merely to host factors but also to environmental factors of etiological significance.

Secondary prevention, which is aimed at remedying as soon as possible the alterable disabilities of the mentally retarded, is a valuable, direct, clinical approach to the reduction of the impairment to a minimum. At the tertiary level of prevention, the sequels that result from neglect or inadequacy of early treatment require major, rehabilitative efforts. All such preventive approaches to the mentally retarded characterize mental health services as distinguished from the more traditional medical services that focus so exclusively on psychopathology and illness that the possibility of offsetting potentialities for healthy development may be overlooked. An inherent feature of mental health practice is the maximizing of both individual endowments and environmental supports such as the psychosocial milieu. The care-giving potentialities of significant persons, of social institutions, and of health, education, and welfare agencies of all kinds are of crucial importance to the mentally retarded. Habilitation and rehabilitation are the major modalities for significantly reducing either the primary or the secondary disabilities of the vast majority of persons who might otherwise be categorized as hopelessly mentally deficient.

THE MEANING OF "INDIRECT" MENTAL HEALTH SERVICES

The significance of the term "indirect" when applied to mental health services can scarcely be overemphasized. The concept of indirect services provides, in fact, a bridge between direct clinical and other care-giving services to the retarded, on the one hand, and the application of the principles of prevention that are embodied in the practice of community psychiatry at its best. Traditionally, the practice of clinical neuropsychiatry in behalf of the mentally retarded has been institutionally oriented; comprehensive services, sometimes of excellent quality and ranging from custodial care to sterilization, have been provided under medical direction in special twenty-four-hour facilities. In those cases for whom no alternative to indefinite hospitalization is warranted, it is entirely appropriate that all of the recipients' needs be met through direct, psychiatric, intramural services. However, most of the mentally retarded do not require hospitalization; wherever they live—with their own families, in foster homes, in residential schools, or in other facilities—it is the nonpsychiatric caregivers who provide the more appropriate direct services, while the community mental health professionals (psychiatrists included) support these efforts as either collaborators, consultants, mental health educators, or developers of community mental health programs for the retarded. The indirect services from psychiatric professionals are not intended to replace the direct, clinical services also needed by the mentally retarded, but rather the consultative, educational, and administrative services of psychiatric and parapsychiatric professionals are intended to enable nonpsychiatric and nonmedical professionals and nonprofessionals to provide what is necessary for the successful habilitation and rehabilitation of the mentally retarded.

In Blain's "zonal" classification of all the people in a given population at risk of mental breakdown, everybody starts out in the prenatal Zone I. While most people are born into Zone II as normally functioning individuals in a normal social milieu, everyone sooner or later gets into trouble, Zone III. The majority of these, with or without outside help, return to Zone II (normality) but some suffer a mental breakdown and move into Zone IV, which Blain identifies as the zone of mental illness. A few mentally retarded are identifiable before birth as existing in Zone I. Most mentally retarded are identified as members of the troubled population of Zone III some years after birth, usually at school age. Some are born into Zone IV, that is, recognizably, severely retarded at birth. The majority, however, in Zone III have the possibility of surmounting their handicaps and with proper help

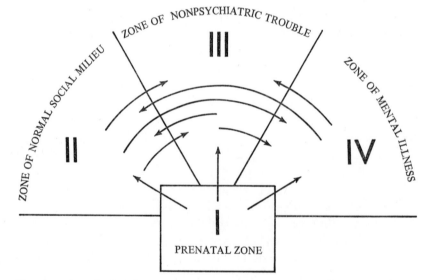

Figure 1. Zonal classification—people. (Blain, Daniel: The organization of psychiatry in the United States. In Arieti, S. (Ed.): *American Handbook of Psychiatry.* New York, Basic Books, 1959, Vol. II, page 1970, courtesy of American Psychiatric Association.)

through the indirect kinds of mental health services may move into the normal Zone II. The less fortunate may, however, end up in Zone IV and require "direct" psychiatric services.

Blain's dynamic concept of the population at risk illustrates how the mentally retarded are actually to be found in any zone. Surely, therefore, they deserve consideration in relationship to their place within the total population rather than being segregated and consigned to separate institutions, partial programs, or unrealistic diagnostic categories. In short, adequate mental health services for the mentally retarded require that they be viewed without prejudice in relationship to the environment which may not only add to their deprivations but may also provide far better mental health services and other resources than traditional policies and practices as yet afford. The mentally retarded deserve consideration as part of the total human community to which comprehensive mental health programs are addressed.

One criterion of comprehensiveness is the inclusion of "indirect" services along with the direct, clinical, and nonclinical services needed by the retarded or any other member of the population at risk of mental breakdown. The point that must never be overlooked is that the primary responsibility for the delivery of mental health services cannot be shirked by mental health professionals. On the other hand, they alone cannot be in direct contact with the population to be reached for purposes of safeguarding everyone's mental health. The mental health specialists, therefore, must work through all those other professionals and nonprofessionals, including the parents of the retarded, who are necessarily in contact, one way or another, with all sectors of the population.

The principal mediators between the mental health professionals and the mentally retarded in any population are either natural parents or foster parents plus a tremendous variety of care-givers or "gate-keepers" in the fields of health, education, and welfare, as well as in industry or any kind of enterprise offering opportunities for employment. The mental health functions of all of these mediators are generally unrecognized, if only for the reason that their primary objectives are not identified with mental health at all. It is not the purpose of the mental health professionals to divert them in any way from their own priorities, but rather merely to make all sorts of nonpsychiatric professionals and non-professionals aware of the mental health components of any enterprise that employs or serves people with a wide range of mental capacities and vulnerabilities.

The ways in which the mental health specialists relate to the mediators referred to above are called "indirect" services, in or-

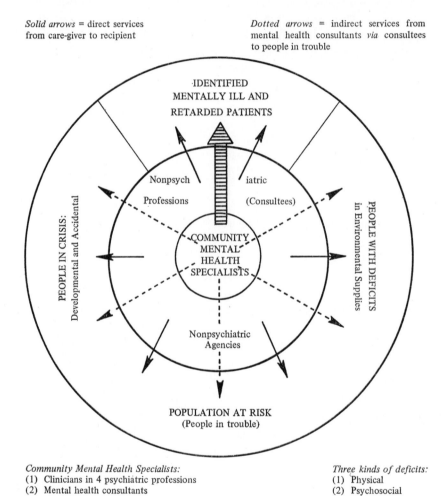

Solid arrows = direct services from care-giver to recipient

Dotted arrows = indirect services from mental health consultants *via* consultees to people in trouble

IDENTIFIED MENTALLY ILL AND RETARDED PATIENTS

Nonpsych / iatric

Professions (Consultees)

PEOPLE IN CRISIS: Developmental and Accidental

PEOPLE WITH DEFICITS in Environmental Supplies

COMMUNITY MENTAL HEALTH SPECIALISTS

Nonpsychiatric Agencies

POPULATION AT RISK (People in trouble)

Community Mental Health Specialists:
(1) Clinicians in 4 psychiatric professions
(2) Mental health consultants
(3) Mental health administrators

Three kinds of deficits:
(1) Physical
(2) Psychosocial
(3) Sociocultural

Figure 2. The human community served directly and indirectly by community mental health specialists.

der to distinguish them from "direct" services in the organization of community mental health programs. Figure 2 depicts this distinction in diagrammatic form.

THEORETICAL CONSIDERATIONS

Caplan's conceptual model of primary prevention[2] is applicable to any kind of mental disorder, including mental retardation. While the epidemiological details of any specific clinical entity are not furnished by Caplan's model, it does offer in a general way the principal, epidemiological considerations which must be taken into account in, not only specific epidemiological studies, but also in conceptualizing the major purposes of a community mental health program. The multifactorial nature of mental disorders is supported by both scientific studies and clinical observations. Indeed, what is most characteristic of American psychiatry is its psychobiological foundations plus its insistence upon consideration of the individual patient in relationship to his total environment. The host factors most pertinent to Caplan's theory are those that are alterable, namely those due to individual history, such as ego-strengths, problem-solving skills, and capacity to tolerate anxiety and frustration. These acquired, alterable factors are the products of the prolonged childhood and adolescence of the human species as contrasted with other mammals. The inalterable host factors depend upon individual fate and include age, sex, and both the socioeconomic class and the ethnic group into which one is born. Between the alterable and the inalterable, there is a set of host factors which may or may not turn out to be alterable, namely, genetic patterns or chromosomal factors.

With respect to environmental factors that hinder or help an individual's ability to adapt or to cope with the vicissitudes of life, Caplan distinguishes between those influences in the community and those environmental forces that on the one hand support or, on the other hand, hinder an individual's personal resistance to mental breakdown or inadequacy. The environmental factors that commonly affect many people to a significant extent within a given community or defined population demand as much attention from mental health professionals as clinicians afford to the idiosyncratic factors that determine a given patient's vulnerabilities.

The approach to the community's role in mental breakdown or inadequacy needs to be twofold: a) from the long-range viewpoint, the environmental factors that mold the development of a person's life-style from birth to death consist of different kinds of "supplies" continually needed by everyone in keeping with his current stage of growth and development; and b) from the short-term viewpoint, attention must be focussed upon two kinds of life-crises, the developmental ones which everybody predictably experiences as well as accidental or unpredictable crises where the stress may precipitate a mental breakdown in even the strongest person.

A CLASSIFICATION OF DIRECT AND INDIRECT MENTAL HEALTH SERVICES

Direct, care-giving services for the mentally retarded include not merely clinical services of a psychiatric, neurological, pediatric, and general medical character, but also nonclinical services such as day-care, education and/or training in special classes or sheltered workshops, plus welfare, guardianship, recreational, and correctional programs geared to the special needs of the retarded, both juvenile and adult. Therefore, a great deal of teamwork between clinical and nonclinical professionals and nonprofessionals is involved. From the point of view of mental health professionals responsible for programs serving the retarded, consequently, direct services are not confined to clinical, psychiatric care but rather consist of collaboration between psychiatric and nonpsychiatric agencies and workers of nonclinical as well as clinical varieties. This state of affairs becomes perfectly obvious when a mental health program for the retarded emerges from institutional settings and provides services in the community.

The essence of true collaboration is that the participating agencies and caregivers retain their respective, autonomous functions; the question of which agency or which worker takes primary responsibility for the mentally retarded recipient is not a question that is determined *a priori* and forever but may, on the contrary, shift with the age as well as the changing mental health needs of the recipient. The collaborators may use one another as specialized consultants and reach working agreements in terms of the recipient's priorities, rather than those of the collaborating professions or agencies. Such collaboration entails both continuous planning on behalf of the mentally retarded individual and constant vigilance lest the recipient become lost in the caseload of one of the collaborating agencies.

This conception of direct, mental health services for the mentally retarded means essentially that the retarded are regarded as joint cases with such changing needs during their lifetimes that no one but a natural parent or legal guardian has permanent responsibility. In practice, there are many difficulties and some hazards to the recipient of collaborative services, to be sure. However, one of the responsibilities of a qualified mental health professional is to see that mental health services for every sector of the population at risk are so organized that all kinds of services are made available in accordance with the needs of the recipients rather than depending upon the convenience or traditions of the providers of services.

In addition to providing direct psychiatric, clinical services on a *solo* basis or in collaboration with other caregivers, the mental health professional serves the mentally retarded indirectly. The organizational functions for the teamwork mentioned above constitute one kind of indirect service. Of equal or greater significance are those indirect services from mental health specialists that consist of consultant-consultee relationships on behalf of the consultee's client, with whom the consultant may never have a direct, face-to-face relationship. For example, as a collaborator, the mental health specialist may provide a psychiatric evaluation by directly examining someone else's client or patient. As a mental health consultant, on the other hand, the mental health specialist's functions are nonclinical and only indirectly benefit the consultee's case. Both consultant and consultee have responsibilities for the mental health of the consultee's client or patient, but the former's responsibility is carried out indirectly through the consultee who works directly with the case, or who is responsible for a nonpsychiatric service to more than one similar case.

The mental health functions of mental health consultants are mainly, but not exclusively, educational in nature. That is to say that the most common function performed by a mental health consultant is to fill in gaps in the knowledge of the consultee that would benefit the case under discussion, or to provide insights that hitherto eluded the consultee. Frequently, however, the consultee is "hung up" on account of acquired, professional attitudes, or because of the customs or rules of the agency in which the consultee works. Such "hang-ups," which are shared by others in the consultee's profession or agency, have to be distinguished from what Caplan calls "Theme-interferences."[2] The latter are individually determined phenomena arising from the unconscious of the consultee. The special technique devised by Caplan to reduce such theme-interferences may be an additional, specialized function of a mental health consultant who has learned the technique.

In addition to consultation about cases of mental retardation, a mental health consultant may be called upon for help regarding the program of an agency, for example, a school system with questions or problems associated with managing educational services to the mentally retarded. Mental health consultation and education, consequently, may take the form of either case consultation or administrative consultation. In both forms, the mental health consultant may be called upon to deal with subject matter that pertains either to the mentally retarded or to the consultees. In other words, case consultation as well as administrative consultation may be case-centered or program-centered, on the one hand, or the consultation may be consultee-centered. In all circumstances, however, the ultimate beneficiary is the mentally retarded individual, which is the reason for calling mental health consultation an indirect service to the retarded.

The mental health functions of the consultees of mental health consultants are different because the consultees retain the responsibility for the direct services to their clients or patients. In general, without going into the particulars for each consultee, the mental health functions of nonpsychiatric agencies and professions are the following: a) provision of the necessary "supplies" mentioned earlier in this chapter; b) manipulation of the environment; c) timely interventions of an extra, supportive nature when life-crises occur; d) case-finding; and e) collaboration with mental health professionals in behalf of joint cases.

A classification of direct and indirect mental health services includes the following items:

A. *Direct Mental Health Services*
    I. In psychiatric settings:
       1. Diagnostic, neuropsychiatric evaluations.
       2. Clinical interventions of a prompt, remedial nature.
       3. Psychiatric rehabilitation.
       4. Any or all of (1) to (3) in collaboration with non-psychiatric clinicians such as pediatricians and nurses.
    II. In nonpsychiatric settings:
       1. Clinical services in collaboration with nonclinical care-givers such as educators, rehabilitation counselors, probation officers assigned to children's protective services, staff on the pediatric or obstetrical services of general hospitals.
       2. Diagnostic, neuropsychiatric evaluations for public agencies such as courts and Medicaid authorities.
B. *Indirect Mental Health Services*
    I. Mental health education:
       1. Community organization of mental health resources in behalf of the mentally retarded.
       2. Public information services to parents' groups, elected officials, volunteers and planning bodies.
       3. On-the-job training in mental health for the staff of agencies in the general fields of health, education, and welfare (tax supported and voluntary).
       4. Preservice educational programs for any care-giving professionals.
    II. Mental health consultation:
       1. Case-consultation to nonpsychiatric professionals (individuals or in groups).
       2. Administrative consultation to nonpsychiatric agencies (individual administrators or staffs).
    III. Collaboration between mental health program administrators and administrators of nonpsychiatric programs with respect to:

1. Conjoint surveying of the unmet mental health needs of the retarded.
2. Priority-setting in meeting needs.
3. Distribution of functions in joint planning.
4. Provision of interagency and interprofessional collaboration on joint cases.
5. Program evaluation.

SUMMARY

Whether or not the mentally retarded, as far as their clinical care is concerned, require direct, clinical, psychiatric services in all cases, is an open question; for some, general medical care may be adequate. The universal need for indirect kinds of mental health services, that is, for preventive services cannot be denied, however. From the point of view of public mental health the responsibility of the psychiatric profession is clear. Furthermore, clinical, psychiatric interventions of a preventive nature, at either the secondary or tertiary levels of prevention, may be essential at critical times. The point has been made that psychiatric collaboration in the care of the mentally retarded is likely to be far more useful in most instances than the traditional, institutionalized, exclusively neuropsychiatric approach whose value to all but the most severely retarded is questionable.

When it comes to the indirect varieties of mental health services, especially those that ensure prevention at the primary level, there are no substitutes for the consultative and educational services provided by mental health specialists from all the major psychiatric professions (psychiatrists, psychiatric nurses and social workers, and clinical psychologists). A failure or inadequacy of psychiatric responsibility in providing such indirect services amounts to abandonment of most of the mentally retarded in a given population at risk.

Community mental health centers and programs claiming to be comprehensive in scope have no grounds for continuing their frequent exclusion of the mentally retarded. Any system for the delivery of public mental health services must be sufficiently flexible and capable of responding realistically to a population that is not merely at risk of mental breakdown in a theoretical sense, but also in a state of flux with respect to both its actual mental health needs and the mental capacities of its members. Institutional models for organizing services have to be abandoned as too rigid. Instead, a system for the delivery of mental health services has to be planned and organized along functional lines with a minimum of structural elements, before it can overcome such rigidities as the segregation of the mentally retarded in the name of giving them special attention. For far too long, the laws and special establishments created for the mentally retarded have had a dehumanizing effect. It is here proposed that the mentally retarded be desegregated through a system of direct and indirect mental health services that brings to bear all appropriate resources in their behalf.

REFERENCES

1. Blain, Daniel: The organization of psychiatry in the United States. In Arieti, S. (Ed.): *American Handbook of Psychiatry*. New York, Basic Books, 1959, Vol. II, pp. 1960-1982.
2. Caplan, Gerald: *Principles of Preventive Psychiatry*. New York, Basic Books, 1964.
3. Caplan, Gerald (Ed.): *Prevention of Mental Disorders in Children*. New York, Basic Books, 1961.
4. Caplan, Gerald: *The Theory and Practice of Mental Health Consultation*. New York, Basic Books, 1970.
5. Hume, Portia Bell: General principles of community psychiatry. In Arieti, S. (Ed.): *American Handbook of Psychiatry*. New York, Basic Books, 1966, Vol. III, pp. 515-541.
6. Hume, Portia Bell: Community psychiatry, social psychiatry, and community mental health work: Some interprofessional relationships in psychiatry and social work. *Am J Psychiatry*, 121:340-343, 1964.
7. Hume, Portia Bell: Social psychiatry as prevention and rehabilitation: Some critical points in evaluation. In Zubin, J. and Frehan, F. A. (Eds.): *Social Psychiatry*. New York, Grune and Stratton, 1968, pp. 300-311.
8. Joint Commission on Mental Health of Children: *Crisis in Child Mental Health: Challenge for the 1970's*. New York, Evanston, and London, Harper and Row, 1970.
9. Katz, Elias: *The Retarded Adult in the Community*. Springfield, Ill., Charles C Thomas, 1968.
10. Lamb, H. Richard, Heath, Don and Downing, Joseph J. (Eds.):

Handbook of Community Mental Health Practice. San Francisco, Jossey-Bass, 1969.

11. Parker, Beulah: *Mental Health Inservice Training: Some Practical Guidelines for the Psychiatric Consultant.* New York, International Universities Press, 1968.
12. Philips, Irving (Ed.): *Prevention and Treatment of Mental Retardation.* New York, Basic Books, 1966.

Chapter 3

PSYCHOTHERAPY WITH BEHAVIORALLY DISTURBED MENTALLY RETARDED

R. K. Janmeja Singh

UNTIL recently there has been a general skepticism about the possibility of psychotherapy for the mentally retarded. Sarason[43] summarizes the reasons for such skepticism as follows:

> The inability of such an individual to control or delay emotional expression, to seek and to accept socially appropriate substitute activities in the face of frustrations and restrictions, to view objectively the behavior of others, to adjust or to want to adjust to the needs of others, to realize the sources and consequences of his behavior—these have been considered the liabilities of the defective individual which make it difficult for him to comprehend and to adjust to the purposes of the psychotherapeutic interview.

Sarason's above quotation implies that much of the behavioral disturbance in the mentally retarded is a direct consequence of his physical condition. This belief is challenged by Heber[24] in his review of research on the personality of the mentally retarded.

This skepticism is the result of a) theoretical approach to understand the personality of the mentally retarded; b) the aims of psychotherapy; and c) the techniques of psychotherapy. Let us take these three aspects one by one.

PERSONALITY OF THE MENTALLY RETARDED

The mentally retarded child is presumably different from an average child in having some neurological and structural defect which is caused by genetic, developmental, or some environmental

NOTE: The author extends his thanks to the following for reading the manuscript and making valuable comments: Dr. John Arsenian, Director of Psychological Research, Boston State Hospital, and Dr. James T. Shelton, Superintendent, Porterville State Hospital.

factors. All mentally retarded are not similar in the extent and nature of their defects. The major part of the following discussion is not applicable to the most profoundly retarded patients. This discussion is an endeavor to understand the personality development of those patients who have sufficient neurological apparatus to present a behavioral problem. If the retardation is due to sociocultural or psychological reasons, then there is hardly any point in belaboring the issue about applicability of psychotherapeutic skills to the treatment of such patients. Psychotherapy may be a useful treatment of choice even with those patients whose retardation is due to neurological or biochemical reasons.

Rappaport[41] states three general points of view in regard to the genesis of behavior disturbance in a brain damaged person.

> The oldest and still most prevalent view attributes the observed thought-disorder and behavioral deviations to irrevocably neural structures (Hunt and Cofer;[27] Klebanoff, Singer, Witlansky[30]). Either impairment in the higher inhibitory cortical centers, or brain-stem lesions are held responsible for hyperactivity, impulsiveness, and hostile or destructive outbursts so commonly found in the brain injured child (Blan;[6] Kahn and Cohen;[29] Strauss and Lehtinen;[50] Timme[52]), and their anxiety is also considered to be determined by the organic lesion (Bender[4]).

The quotation from Sarason fits in with such an approach.

> The second view in general leaves a hiatus between the organic and the psychological factors, the implication being that the former are irreparable and can only be controlled by means of drugs and/or by delimitations of the environment to make it nonfrustrating. As for the psychological factors, this view advises guidance of the parents and treating the "accompanying neurotic problems" of the child (Bender,[4] Bradley,[7] Weil[54]).

> According to the third view, the total picture presented is the result of the interaction of functional and organic factors (Bettelheim and Hartmann[5]). Indeed, in restating Schilder's position, Rapaport[40] (pp. 660, 285) has suggested that organic damage and psychological disturbance may use the same mechanisms, though differing in intensity and extent. The mechanisms referred to are the ego functions. Whether symptoms are characteristic of brain damage, of psychological disturbance, or of both present simultaneously, they still involve the ego functions.

The author subscribes to the third point of view in general. He has attempted to study the personality of the mentally retarded within a psychodynamic frame of reference. He has observed that there is no such single entity as the personality of the mentally retarded. The range of personality patterns and behavior disorders is as varied in the mentally retarded as it is in a population with average intelligence. One can find all sorts of disorders ranging from schizophrenic to neurotic problems of bed wetting, sexual perversions, and sociopathic behavior disorders. The author has found one study explicitly designed to explore the nature of behavior disorders in mentally retarded. Jolles[31] (p. 35) studied thirty-four mentally retarded children by using the Rorschach personality test. "He discovered twenty-one cases of anxiety neuroses, six schizophrenic personalities, one depressive, and one character neurosis."

The mentally retarded differs from the general population in the functioning of his ego apparatus. He still has similar instinctual needs. There are some exceptions, e.g. profoundly retarded cases. He still grows in an environment and he has parents and siblings. However, all parents do not react to mental retardation in the same way and the environmental interaction is not at all identical. This may be why one does not find a single personality pattern in the mentally retarded. Because the personality of a mentally retarded child is the result of a variety of interactions between internal and external environment and is not just a result of his neurological defects, it would seem plausible to endeavor to change the behavior by means of psychotherapeutic interaction. If we believe that the behavior disorder is entirely a *direct* consequence of neurological damage, then only neurological therapy could be expected to help.

AIMS OF PSYCHOTHERAPY

The statement that mental retardation is incurable is misunderstood. It should not be used to mean that psychotherapeutic process is meant to raise the IQ. The primary aim of psychotherapy is not to raise the intellectual functioning. It is obvious that one cannot cure by psychotherapy the physical and neurological defects of the mentally retarded. Psychotherapy does not aim to make a genius of an average person. The aim of psychotherapy is to deal with the behavior disorders and the crippling effects of emotional conflicts. Nevertheless, it is possible that a person might be able to function better intellectually as a result of psycho-therapy because ego resources are liberated from the instinctual interference and the sphere of conflict-free ego is extended.

A second question may be raised regarding the effectiveness of psychotherapy in making an individual capable of "independent social" existence. It is pointed out that the mentally retarded by definition[12, 43] is a socially inadequate person. It may be so when one thinks of society at large where the individual is expected to earn an independent living, indulge in competition, etc. Society cannot always protect a less intelligent person from the stressful elements inherent in it. One can look at it from a slightly different angle. Society itself is differentiated into different subdivisions and a person who fits in one circle of society may be a complete failure in another. Everyone "structures" his society according to his potential and needs, and his happiness lies in *how he adjusts to his society.*

Similarly, society also has children who need adult protection and guidance but there are only some children who need psychotherapy to adjust to their role as children.

Now let us assume that the mentally retarded need a protective environment because of their low mental functioning. This limited environment is their sub-society. They have to adjust to it and also make an adjustment and to realize the place of this sub-society in the total society. In this society also there are rules, there are ambitions, there are people who are involved in the care of these patients, and there are parents and friends who come to visit. The adjustment to this environment is also difficult and raises problems. Psychotherapy can help in improving this adjustment for those who may have to accept this environment all their lives. There are others, however, who might be able to make adjustments to society away from this protective environment. There are many borderline, mildly or moderately retarded, patients who might make some adjustment in a less protective environment if they did not present behavior problems.

Michal-Smith[34] discusses the realistic limitation of the psychiatric time available for such purposes and the expected returns. Even in that light it seems worthwhile to do intensive psychotherapy with the mentally retarded. Not only does it make the patient more comfortable with himself (which could in itself be sufficient reason) and the total environment of a hospital, family care, or his own family a more cheerful place to live, it also is more economical. There will be less staff needed for the care of these patients if there are less behaviorally disturbed children and there will be less destruction of materials. It will reduce the emotional stress and interference in the lives of the families of the retarded. In the case of the mentally retarded we can consider what society might save economically and what he could provide toward the emotional well-being of people around him.

There is another very important reason that warrants psychotherapy with the mentally retarded. It is very difficult to differentiate between the truly retarded who has some neurological or structural defect and the person whose mental functioning is retarded because of some severe emotional disturbance. Sarason has rightly challenged the diagnosis of mental retardation in the cases of those patients who improved significantly in their intellectual functioning after they had been in psychotherapy. For this reason he has recommended psychotherapy as an essential tool to differentiate the functional retardation from organic retardation. Those who work in the hospitals for the mentally retarded frequently find cases where the patient was committed to the hospital for the mentally retarded diagnosed as an organic when actually the etiology was functional. More attention to the psychological needs of the mentally retarded patients would eliminate loss of time and produce rich rewards in terms of better emotional adjustment and possible realization of the patient's potentialities.

PSYCHOTHERAPEUTIC APPROACH

Michal-Smith quotes from Freud's lecture before the College of Physicians in Vienna in 1904. In discussing the conditions under which psychotherapy was contraindicated Freud said the following:

> Those patients who do not possess a reasonable degree of education and reliable character should be refused. The qualification which is the determining factor of fitness for psychoanalytic treatment is whether the patient is educable. To be quite safe, we should limit our choice of patients to those who possess a normal mental con-

dition, since in the psychoanalytic method this is used as a foothold from which to obtain control of the morbid manifestations.

Hutt[28] alludes to the skepticism expressed by Rogers and Fenichel. Rogers believes that the subject must have adequate capacities for dealing with life situations and that he must have at least dull normal intelligence to profit from psychotherapy. Fenichel states that the mentally retarded individual cannot profit from psychoanalysis since the ego does not have the capacity to face its conflicts. "However, even though Fenichel rules out the use of psychoanalysis with mentally retarded individuals, he states that such persons might respond to psychoanalytically oriented psychotherapy."[28] Sarason, along with others, points out the fact that many of the retarded patients are not verbal. Lack of verbal skills, they point out, rules out psychotherapy as an effective tool.

All of the above mentioned comments look extreme and some of these are based upon inferences drawn from working with the intellectually normal populations. Moreover, psychotherapy and psychoanalysis seemed to be used interchangeably, which is questionable.

Since 1904, there had been revolutionary developments in the theory of psychoanalysis. The emergence of ego psychology* has changed the whole emphasis in psychoanalytic theory and these developments are most useful and relevant in understanding the personality of the mentally retarded. As Hartmann[22] has pointed out, it is particularly the study of ego functions that might facilitate the meeting between the psychoanalytic and the neurophysiologic approaches.

In psychoanalytic treatment and practice there have been equally revolutionary developments. The psychoanalytic study of children especially has opened many doors for the development of new techniques. Traditional psychoanalysis is not the only method of treatment. At present the analyst has much more understanding of personality dynamics and is better equipped to understand and work through behavior problems than he was sixtyseven years ago. It is not necessary for the children to verbalize. The analyst uses play or painting as a medium of communication and helps the children to work through their problems.

---

* See references: 16-18, 22, 31, 36-39, 44.

Melanie Klein equates the play of children with the free associations of adult patients under analysis. Anna Freud sees it as a dream representation of unconscious conflicts. In either case, play is used to understand the psychodynamics of the child and the therapeutic process develops even though the child is unable to verbalize his thoughts and feelings. A trained analyst attempts to understand the patient through the symbolic representations of his thought processes. The author does not mean to suggest that an adult with a mental age of a child is similar to the child in his personality functioning. Instead, there is a vast difference. Although the intellectual level may be the same, the adult differs in the nature and intensity of his impulses and his physical capacities. But the nonverbal techniques which are developed by working with children can be successfully utilized with adults with poor verbal and mental abilities.

Moreover, the talking in adult psychotherapy serves a purpose similar to playing and painting for children. Talking during the transference situation is more a concealed representation of the feelings and fears aroused in relation to the therapist. The therapist has to be perceptive of the unconscious fantasies of the patient by inferring from the manifest content of the verbalizations during the therapy hour and interpreting the unconscious significance of such verbalizations. It is very similar to the interpretation of play, dream, or paintings. In this way the verbal medium of communication is only one of the several media of communication of unconscious dynamics. Psychotherapy is not solely dependent upon the ability to verbalize.

The role of the intellect has also been greatly overemphasized in the psychotherapeutic process. The development of personality is not a conscious intellectual process. On the other hand, there are some fantasies aroused in relation to the instinctual needs and these might be accompanied by certain fears, guilt, or apprehensions caused by the environmental conditions. The child does not develop conflicts consciously, nor does a normal child resolve such conflicts by conscious efforts. The unconscious conflicts manifest themselves in adult behavior if they have not been resolved because of some unusual events in the *psychological environment* of the child. Presumably, the patient brings up these unconscious instinctual needs and the fears associated with them in the transference situation. If the transference develops to the extent that the repressed impulses are aroused but the fears associated with the impulse do not come true, then this in itself is therapeutic (corrective emotional experience). The generalization value of the fears and guilt associated with the impulses is greatly reduced. There is a deconditioning of the fear or guilt response even if the person may not become "aware" of the original conditioning situation. Intellectual discussion may be unnecessary.

In this light "insight" does not necessarily have to be an intellectual process. If it were so then the obsessive-compulsive patient could be said to have complete insight. But his talking about his murderous thoughts is no more an insight than is the hysterics' talking of their paralyses. The obsessive-compulsive verbalizations about his thoughts and actions are just the statements of his symptoms. He has little "insight" into the unconscious conflicts that led up to his symptomatology in thought and action, as does the hysterical patient. It takes much more time and effort to bring about the integration of thought and affects in an obsessive-compulsive than in a hysteric. For a profitable therapeutic relationship one has to get affectively involved before he can see the reality of his fears associated with instinctual demands.

"Insight" as used to describe a therapeutic phenomenon is more a corrective emotional experience than the intellectual understanding of one's psychodynamics. If insight is predominantly an emotional experience then the emphasis which is placed on the intellectual abilities of the patients is unwarranted.

If a patient has the potential to get caught in a conflict, the same potential can be used to reduce that conflict. Moreover, in psychotherapeutic process the first step is the way the patient structures the therapy relationship. He brings to the therapy situation his unique ways of relating to people and handling his impulses when they are aroused. The therapist, instead of reacting to the patient's unrealistic demands and fears, makes him realize the unreality of his attitudes which were aroused in relation to the therapist. It is a twofold process.

First, the patient expresses his impulses and conflicts verbally and/or nonverbally in the transference situation. His fears associated with his impulses are aroused but if the therapist is still accepting, his fears do not come true. This type of experience repeated enough in itself reduces the intensities of anxieties and helps reduction of conflicts and constraints on ego functioning.

Second and ideally, the therapist does not stop there. After the patient realizes the unreality of his behavior and attitudes in relation to the therapist and begins to feel comfortable with his immediate conflicts, the therapist moves a step further, i.e. tries to clarify the real object person to whom they belong. This is done by interpreting the manifest content and trying to discover in what role the patient was perceiving the therapist, which led up to his reactions during that particular time of therapy. Suppose that these were the abnormal fears in relation to the father figure. There is still the problem of what aspect of father's "perceived" behavior gave rise to such emotional attitudes. Furthermore, how and under what conditions his perceptions got distorted and his emotional attitudes were formed which affects his present behavior. In short, one can go from the immediate to the past in an attempt to trace the original conditioning experiences by understanding and interpreting the defenses, conflicts and impulses as they emerge in the therapy situation. But this is an ideal which is seldom possible and *in most cases may not be desirable or needed to deal with the present behavior problem.* Especially in the case of the mentally retarded there is not a very highly developed neurological apparatus and, therefore, their psychodynamics are more obvious and more amenable to change under proper therapeutic circumstances and corrective emotional experiences.

Psychotherapeutic intervention brings about behavioral change. The changes in the patient and the meaning of his behavior have to be *emotionally* understood by those persons who are significantly involved with the patient, such as parents[21] and other professionals working with the retarded. Mental health consultation should be made available[45, 46] to these persons simultaneously with the treatment of the patient.

Lastly, it may be pointed out that the range of retardation and physical and neurological handicap is great and psychotherapy techniques have to be devised according to the degree of fantasy life and ideation present in the child. If a child has fantasy enough to be afraid, depressed, or angry it is quite plausible to work through his problems by psychotherapy. If the neurological and structural damage is so great that the patient responds only at a reflex level, even then simple conditioning techniques might be tried to change an undesirable reflex behavior.

The present-day behavior modification techniques[2] have been very profitably used in bringing about behavioral changes in the mentally retarded.

REFERENCES

1. Abel, T.: Resistance and difficulties in the psychotherapy of mental retardates. *J Clin Psychol,* 9:107-109, 1953.
2. Anant, Santokh S. (Ed.): The use of operant conditioning with the mental retardates: A report of a pilot experiment. In *Readings in Behavior Therapies.* New York, MSS Educational Publishing Company, Inc., 1969.
3. Beier, E. G., Garlaw, L., and Stacey, C. L.: The fantasy life of the mental defective. *Am J Ment Defic,* 55:582-589, 1951.
4. Bender, L.: Psychological problems of children with organic brain disease. *Am J Orthopsychiatry,* 29, 1949.
5. Bettelheim, S. and Hartmann, H.: On parapraxes in the korsakaw psychosis. In Rapaport, D. (Ed.): *Organization and Pathology of Thought.* New York, Columbia University Press, 1959.
6. Blan, A.: Mental changes following head trauma in children. *Arch Neurol,* 35, 1935.
7. Bradley, C.: Organic factors in the psychopathology of childhood. In Hoch, P. H. and Zubin, J. (Eds.): *Psychopathology of Childhood.* New York, Grune and Stratton, 1953.
8. Burton, A.: Psychotherapy with the mentally retarded. *Am J Ment Defic,* 58:485-489, 1954.
9. Chidester, L. and Menninger, K.: The application of psychoanalytic methods to the study of mental retardation. *Am J Orthopsychiatry,* 6:616-625, 1936.
10. Clark, L. P.: *The Nature and Treatment of Amentia.* London, Brailliere, Tindall and Cox, 1933.
11. Cobb, S.: Personality as affected by lesions of the brain. In Hunt, J. McV. (Ed.): *Personality and the Behavior Disorders.* New York, Ronald Press, 1944, Vol. 2.
12. Doll, E. A.: The essentials of an inclusive concept of mental deficiency. *Am J Ment Defic,* 46:214-219, 1941.
13. Doll, E. A.: Definition of mental deficiency. *Train Sch Bull,* 37:153-159, 1941.

14. Fenichel, O.: *The Psychoanalytic Theory of Neuroses.* New York, W. W. Norton and Company, Inc., 1945.
15. Foale, M.: The special difficulties of the high grade mental defective adolescent. *Am J Ment Defic,* 60:867-877, 1956.
16. Freud, S.: *Beyond the Pleasure Principle.* New York, Liveright, 1942.
17. Freud, S.: *The Ego and the Id.* New York, W. W. Norton and Company, Inc., 1961.
18. Freud, S.: Formulations Regarding the Two Principles in Mental Functioning. In *Collected Papers of Sigmund Freud,* Vol. IV. London, Hogarth, 1946.
19. Glassman, L.: Is dull normal intelligence a contraindication for psychotherapy? *Smith College Studies in Social Work,* 13:275-298, 1945.
20. Gunzburg, H. C.: Psychotherapy with the feeble-minded. In Clarke, Ann M. and Clarke, A. D. B. (Eds.): *Mental Deficiency: The Changing Outlook.* New York, The Free Press, 1965.
21. Hart, Wayne: Psychiatric management of the mentally retarded child. In Poser, Charles M. (Ed.): *Mental Retardation: Diagnosis and Treatment.* New York, Harper and Row, 1969.
22. Hartmann, H.: Ego Psychology and the Problem of Adaptation. In Rapaport, D. (Ed.): *Organization and Pathology of Thought.* New York, Columbia University Press, 1959.
23. Healy, V. and Bronner, A. F.: *Treatment and What Happened Afterward.* Boston, Judge Baker Guidance Center, 1939.
24. Heber, Rick: Personality. In Stevens, Harvey A. and Heber, Rick (Eds.): *Mental Retardation: A Review of Research.* Chicago, The University of Chicago Press, 1964.
25. Heiser, K. F.: Psychotherapy in a residential school for mentally retarded children. *Train Sch Bull,* 50:211-218, 1954.
26. Humphreys, E. J.: Investigative psychiatry in the field of mental deficiency as shown by the Proceedings of the American Association on Mental Deficiency. *Proceedings of the American Association in Mental Deficiency,* 40:195-206, 1935.
27. Hunt, J. McV. and Cofer, C. N.: Psychological Deficit. In Hunt, J. McV. (Ed.): *Personality and the Behavior Disorders, II.* New York, Ronald Press, 1944.
28. Hutt, M. L. and Gibby, R. G.: *The Mentally Retarded Child.* Boston, Allyn and Bacon, Inc., 1958.
29. Kahn, E. and Cohen, L. C.: Organic driveness: a brain system syndrome and an experience. *New Eng J Med,* 210, 1939.
30. Klebanoff, S. C., Singer, J. L., and Witlansky, H.: Psychological consequences of brain lesions and ablations. *Psychol Bull,* 51, 1959.
31. Kris, E.: On preconscious mental processes. In Rapaport, D. (Ed.): *Organization and Pathology of Thought.* New York, Columbia University Press, 1959.

32. Leichner, Abraham M.: Observations on individual and group counseling of the individual with cerebral palsy. *Child,* 23:305-352, 1957.
33. McLachlan, D. G.: Emotional aspects of the backward child. *Am J Ment Defic,* 60:323-330, 1955.
34. Michal-Smith, H. and Kastein, S.: *The Special Child: Diagnosis, Treatment, and Habilitation.* Seattle, Washington, New School for the Special Child, Inc., 1962.
35. Philips, Irving (Ed.): *Prevention and Treatment of Mental Retardation.* New York, Basic Books, Inc., 1966. (Chapters 9 and 14.)
36. Piaget, J.: Principal factors determining intellectual education from childhood to adult life. *Harvard Tercentenary.* Cambridge, Massachusetts, Harvard University Press, 1937.
37. Piaget, J.: The biological problem of intelligence. In Rapaport, D. (Ed.): *Organization and Pathology of Thought.* New York, Columbia University Press, 1959.
38. Rapaport, D.: A historical survey of psychoanalytic ego psychology. *Bull Philadelphia Assoc Psychoanal,* 8:105-120, 1958.
39. Rapaport, D.: Toward a theory of thinking. In Rapaport, D. (Ed.): *Organization and Pathology of Thought.* New York, Columbia University Press, 1959.
40. Rapaport, D.: *Organization and Pathology of Thought.* New York, Columbia University Press, 1959.
41. Rappaport, S. R.: Behavior disorders and ego development in a brain injured child. *Psychoanal Study Child,* 16:423-449, 1961.
42. Rogers, C. R.: *Counseling and Psychotherapy.* New York, Houghton Mifflin Company, 1942.
43. Sarason, S. B.: *Psychological Problems in Mental Deficiency.* New York, Harper and Brothers, 1959.
44. Schilder, P.: Studies concerning the psychology and symptomatology of general paresis. In Rapaport, D. (Ed.): *Organization and Pathology of Thought.* New York, Columbia University Press, 1959.
45. Singh, R. K. J., Tarnower, William, and Chen, Ronald: *Community Mental Health Consultation and Crisis Intervention.* Berkeley, California, Book People, 1971.
46. Singh, R. K. J.: *Developing Community Mental Health Services and Skills.* Chicago, Aldine-Atherton, Inc. (In preparation.)
47. Solnit, A. J. and Stark, M. N.: Mourning and the birth of a defective child. *Psychoanal Study Child,* 16:523-536, 1961.
48. Stacey, L. V. and Demartino, M. F.: *Counseling and Psychotherapy With Mentally Retarded.* Glencoe, Illinois, The Free Press, 1957, Chapter 4.
49. Stephens, E.: Defensive reactions of mentally retarded adults. *Social Casework,* 34:119-124, 1953.

50. Strauss, A. A. and Lehtinen, L. E.: *Psychopathology and Education of the Brain Injured Child.* New York, Grune and Stratton, 1947.
51. Thorne, F. C.: Counseling and psychotherapy with mental defectives. *Am J Ment Defic,* 52:263-271, 1948.
52. Timme, A. R.: What has neurology to offer child guidance? *Neurology II,* 2:435-440, 1952.
53. Tredgold, A. F.: *A Textbook of Mental Deficiency.* Baltimore, Maryland, William Wood and Company, 1937, p. 4.
54. Weil, A. P.: *Seminar.* Philadelphia, Institute of Philadelphia Association for Psychoanalysis, 1958.

Chapter 4

PSYCHOTHERAPEUTIC CONSIDERATIONS WITH MENTALLY RETARDED AND DEVELOPMENTALLY DISABLED CHILDREN

Henry Leland and Daniel E. Smith

THE mentally retarded child who demonstrates sufficient maladaptive behavior, that a community mental health facility is sought for help, needs the type of treatment usually included under the rubrics of psychotherapy or play therapy. In this chapter we will discuss some of the broad implications of the concept of therapy with the mentally retarded as it applies to children who have to be helped to modify behaviors which make their survival in the community or in the home otherwise untenable. We will outline some of the broad principles of play therapy based on our previous book.[7] We will also review some of the more recent developments related to problems of delivery of services, manpower, and types of children to be served. These new developments concern moving away from the doctor-patient service model in favor of work with groups of individuals and the utilization of different types of professional and subprofessional personnel. And finally, we will discuss some of the factors relating to the child in the home, recognizing that if we are to be successful in our efforts to modify the behavior of retarded children, the utilization of the concept of a total milieu must be applied to such a program.

Our approach is essentially threefold. *First,* there is an unwritten law that the less able the child is to function or to evolve the appropriate coping skills when left to his own devices, the greater is the need for directed intervention. We are not interested in becoming involved in a theoretical discussion of the values of non-

38

directive, cathartic or other forms of free play. Rather we have to recognize that the mentally retarded child has a great deal of difficulty in utilizing the cues and stimuli of the surrounding environment and that this difficulty creates very real problems in his overall need to make appropriate coping decisions.[4] It is this failure to make appropriate coping decisions that probably leads to his having come to the attention of the clinic in the first place, i.e. the child who gets included in play therapy or any form of psychological intervention has usually already demonstrated a number of coping failures within his community.

The various community resources represented by clinical services are typically the last resort of a parent in attempting to deal with the problem behavior of their child. Thus, the clinical situation has to deal not only with a child who is demonstrating maladaptive behavior and inappropriate coping responses, but one who has been demonstrating such behaviors over a period of time and already has a history of failure experiences and inappropriate social interaction. In the face of this history it would be difficult to expect that the child could, with those disabilities, freely come into a therapeutic situation and be able to develop insight into his problems. Such ability would imply that he was aware of what he was doing or could easily, on his own resources, become aware; this would be inconsistent with the diagnosis of mental retardation. If the child is considered retarded and behaves in that manner, it is not appropriate to expect that he would gain awareness of his behaviors, primarily because he has had no history of success experiences. Therefore, if he is to gain understanding, it must come through the therapeutic process and the more retarded the child appears in the therapy sessions, the greater the amount of directed play and directed intrusions which must come from the therapists.

A *second* major principle is, regardless of what the therapist feels about social standards, cultural mores, etc., the particular differences that are present in the child's environment cannot be expected to be carried by him as his personal cross. Rather, the child, because of his retardation, must be brought to a level which will permit him to live in his environment regardless of its nature. The therapist does not attempt to remake the child in his own image, and in fact, has a major responsibility not to introduce so many new variables (even though they may be considered positive in the broad sense of social standards), that the child will be unable to interact appropriately with his own family or within the social environment in which he has to live. The therapist must have cognizance of the social forces present in the community from which the child derives and must avoid disrupting the social ecology of the child in introducing the behavior modification processes required. Again, it must be recognized that the child was not surviving properly or he would not have been brought for clinical services. On the other hand, the need for modification may be nowhere as great as the therapist might expect in terms of standard mores. Rather, some relatively simple behaviors might have to be modified which would permit the child to go forward in his personal environment without a tremendously complicated therapy program. In this regard, play therapy does not have to be considered a long-term, highly involved procedure but may be a relatively short-term, simple procedure, leading to the modification of one or two very specific behaviors which are causing the child a great deal of difficulty.

Third, it is recognized that children tend to learn primarily from each other and the processes of imitation may be as valuable as the intervention of the therapist. Therefore, much of the modification may occur better within groups of children than on an individual basis. There are instances when a more individual approach might be valuable. We have come to feel, as we will discuss below, that some of the better play therapy concepts involve a mixture of individual and group approaches, including possibly multiple therapists at varying levels of professional training.

MANIPULATION OF STRUCTURE

When we evolve methods of modifying existing behavior or when we develop procedures for new behavioral functions, the atmosphere of the therapeutic setting and the attitudes of the therapists reveal themselves to be extremely important in the conditioning processes we are trying to establish. This general idea is best represented by the concept of structure. The presence or absence of an organized system of therapeutic procedures becomes literally the keystone of the whole therapeutic process. Where there is a tightly organized, well-developed system of procedures and methods, we would say that this process is highly structured. Where there is a less developed system, not as well organized, and where the methods of procedures are not strictly followed, we would say that this is lacking in structure or to use the terminology we are employing, unstructured. We would define structure as the degree of preconception of form or order found in the therapeutic field.

We are saying that the key to the psychotherapeutic process with retarded children is the modification of behavior, and the key to the modification of behavior is the manipulation and control of the structure or the order and form that surround the child during the therapeutic process. We are not implying that this is the only way to modify behavior, but insofar as we are dealing with that aspect of retarded behavior related to coping and thus that aspect which is tied into both cognition and learning, we find that the amount of organization and form which a therapist must use is very closely related to the level of behavior which requires modification.

Manipulation of structure thus becomes more than just a manipulation of the child's therapeutic milieu. What is attempted in the therapy situation, that which makes it therapy rather that just another behavior modification process, is that the child is put into the kinds of life situations which are causing him the greatest difficulty with his adaptive behavior. The recommendation for psychotherapy grows out of his behavior and not out of a vague group of emotional patterns or diagnostic labels. A child should not be recommended for psychotherapy because he is described as aggressive or acting out or some other such pattern, nor because he would be described as psychoneurotic or schizophrenic. Rather, he should be recommended for psychotherapy because there are certain specific behaviors which he manifests regularly when faced with certain kinds of environmental stimuli. These behaviors disturb the surrounding environment and thus make the child extremely visible in that environment and subject to pressures to remove him from that environment. It is the role of the therapist to try to determine what these specific behaviors are, what specific cognitive style the child uses in attempting to cope with these environmental stimuli recognizing that the particular coping model which the child evolves is also a part of his mental retardation.

When the therapist is able to determine what behaviors seem to be the key sources of the environmental upsets surrounding the child and when he is also able to determine the child's level of development, both socially and intellectually, and the child's level of previous training and experience, it is possible for the therapist to establish a pattern of approach which will take these factors as a guide for the therapeutic procedure. The therapist attempts to set up situations most consistent with the developmental and experiential level of the child and he attempts a structure which will force the child to modify the behavioral modes which are causing the difficulty and will give cues and guides as to what different types of behavioral modes might be attempted to better deal with the situation.

Recognizing that one of the key elements of reward in the therapy situation is the child's ability to maintain social permission to carry out behaviors of his own choice, the question of manipulating structure centers around how much the child is to be rewarded with permission for certain behaviors and how much he is to be punished by having these behaviors blocked. Thus, if the child has a mode of coping with environmental needs which is inconsistent with the expectations and critical demands of his social milieu then these behaviors must be stopped. If this particular mode continues the therapist must interfere with the child's choice of behavior, must intrude upon the child until the child, in order to avoid this intrusion, is willing to modify his behavior. However, if the mode of coping that the child chooses in relationship to the therapeutic situation is consistent with the critical demands of society, then the therapist rewards him by permitting him to continue and thus gives him a sense of self-concept in that he has freely chosen a behavioral mode which may be rewarded instead of being intruded upon.

Much of this approach to play therapy centers around the ability of the retarded child to utilize environmental cues appropriately and to make social decisions based on these cues. This is an area which yields itself readily to training and is an area where reversal of the retarded behavior is to be generally expected. One does not use the same therapeutic process with all retarded children, but rather modifies the type of process along the lines of the amount of structure to be introduced, dependent on the needs of these children. We have arranged these into four general areas.* Children with different types of coping problems have to have a different type of therapeutic approach and a single concept of play therapy cannot be utilized generally.

This overview of the concept of manipulation of structure in the play therapeutic process has attempted to show that one of the major bases for psychotherapy with the mentally retarded is their demonstrated inability to cope successfully with the social and natural demands of their environment. The function of play therapy thus becomes a form of reeducation of modes of adaptation which are considered to be a reversible aspect of mental retardation.[6] However, the play therapeutic process must be modified in terms of developmental needs of the patient and this seems to be best accomplished by dealing either with the level of structure found in the various materials utilized in play therapy or in the amount of organization and preconception associated with the therapist himself. If these factors are taken into consideration, there is a strong possibility of behavioral shaping and modification on a relatively short-term basis. Specific behaviors which violate the critical demands of the child's environment can be changed. In the long run, such therapeutic processes, while not dealing with labels such as neurotic and schizophrenic, nonetheless make the retarded child a more livable person and more able to remain in the community.

GOALS AND PROCEDURES

The goals of play therapy with retarded children are varied but they generally center around attempts to raise the level of functioning and to control behavior. It is hoped that the child will learn to do more things, to improve his ability and, through increased ability, to deal with critical situations, so that he will be

---

* A thorough discussion of this approach to the therapeutic process appears in Leland and Smith (1965). What appears here is a brief overview.

happier and a more useful person. There are differences in opinion but in general we can say that any planned or "goal directed" attempt to create behavioral change, as long as an effort has been made to establish a close interpersonal relationship between the patient and the therapist, as long as an effort has been made to create an organized treatment setting, and as long as the processes of communication are emphasized, should be considered psychotherapy. Differences in materials and differences in procedures will produce a different type of therapeutic result.

The personality changes sought in the retarded individual are those which will make him more able to conform to the demands of the community. He should be able to take from his environment, as does the normal child, the cues to guides to learning in both the behavioral and intellectual spheres. Questions on standard psychometric scales request information, which in terms of standardization the child must have before he enters school. He could learn it in school but he should have that information under his control before he enters into any kind of formal learning situation. This knowledge has to come to him from his milieu. It may have been presented by television, by overheard remarks, by logic, etc., but whatever the source, the milieu has produced sufficient cues that he knows, for example, that a dog has four legs, though no one has upended a dog and explained it to him. The retarded child seems to be blocked in this area. He does not draw on the information which the culture provides. Everything he knows he has had to learn either through very arduous struggle or by having it taught to him in a very painstaking manner—usually through a process which involves conditioning. The reasons for this blockage are varied. Regardless of the cause, the result is that the child's functional level has been lowered by his inability to use minimal cues to guide him to the expected behavior.

When the child seems to be an "invisible" part of the surrounding community, he is accepted for himself at whatever level he functions, and is not constantly being made aware of his mental deficiency. He seems to be able to develop a suitable adjustment. Some children break down later, in adult life, due to changes in social relationships, but this is easier to handle if as a child there was a sense of belonging. The child who is not able to feel that he is part of the day-to-day world, who feels that he has nothing to say about his future but is in the hands of forces which are both frightening and out of his area of control, becomes disturbed and needs special treatment over and above the processes utilized to deal with his abnormal level of mental development.

The behavior changes in which we are most interested are related to the development of a consciousness of social stimuli and an ability, once the child is aware of these stimuli, to modify his own processes in keeping with them. This produces a pattern of behavior which is both socially acceptable and personally rewarding. There is no easy formula because children have different demands and requirements based on their own self-concept, the image they have of themselves, the image they have of the people around them, their families, their friends, their peers, etc., as well as the rest of their life experiences.

The psychotherapy goals for the mental subnormal are those which tend to accelerate his ability to mature and to learn. It is the need for acceleration which becomes one of the most important problems because there is a backlog of decelerated learning which has to be overcome. We need ways of replacing faulty learning and conditioning new learning. This can be accomplished if the therapist is aware of the principles of how children learn. He can arrange his therapy procedure and therapeutic approach in keeping with the growth and developmental patterns of his patient or group of patients and thus be in a position to accelerate these growth patterns. The child must constantly be aware of what he is doing in the play session and be willing to indicate his awareness by either responding to the therapist actively or behaving in a manner that indicates this awareness has been achieved. This requires an emphasis on cognitive processes. The child has to intellectualize his behavior in order to achieve recognition and approbation from his therapist. The process can be described as *forcing the child to think*. Therefore, besides the freedom from intolerable disappointment, which the psychotherapeutic process should represent to the retarded child, it must also represent an introduction to social and individual responsibility. If the child behaves in a more socially acceptable way he is less likely to run into disappointments than if he behaves in a less socially acceptable way. With this realization comes improved cognition and with improved cognition higher functioning. Thus, the technique of *"forcing the child to think"* becomes a way of accelerating cognitive growth and developmental processes. There may be instances where the child is overly resistant to this approach and in those cases additional modes of intrusion must be sought.

Part of the maladaption is the child's general lack of understanding that rules and regulations are not aimed specifically at him, but rather the needs of the social order. He must realize that when he is bawled out for stepping into the street rather than waiting at a stop sign, or looking for cars, this is not a personal rejection or attack but rather is the way society functions so both pedestrians and cars can exist in the same world. For this reason the therapist has a responsibility for establishing limits. Limits must be conceived *first* in terms of the relationship of the patient to the therapist (this may reach the point of personal safety); *second,* they must be related to the relationship of the patient to materials utilized in the play; and *third,* they must be related to the time and place (setting). These limits are however, in a broader sense, most related to the child's gaining understanding that in spite of the fact that the therapist has imposed limits, the child is still accepted, he is still "loved" by the therapist and these limits are not put on him as a way of punishing him but rather as a way of increasing his freedom within the therapy situation.

Concerning the third type of limits (time and place) there are some additional factors. "Time" refers to the limits set on the therapy session. Here we have inescapable limits in the sense that time passes regardless of what else occurs. This can be used to help the child realize that there are many forces in nature or things in society which, as far as he is concerned, are immutable. However, he finds that though unchangeable, it nonetheless provides continuity and thus while it stops one session, it also starts the next.

"Place" refers to the playroom or play therapy setting and it is considered a limit in the sense that it is usually the only place that the child interacts with the therapist as a *therapist*. Both the child and the therapist must be aware of the special roles and relationships the setting provides. Thus, some things are possible in the play room that are not permitted outside. The playroom becomes the source of freedom for the child and the therapist helps him use this freedom constructively. For this reason we have suggested that "dirty" activities (e.g. games, trucks) be done in a different room. Also, the room and the therapist become united in the child's mind and they come to symbolize both the freedom of activity and the source of models.

TYPES OF PLAY THERAPY

The four different types of play therapy we use are the following: a) unstructured materials with unstructured therapeutic approaches (U-U); b) unstructured materials with structured therapeutic approaches (U-S); c) structured materials with unstructured approaches (S-U); d) structured materials with structured therapeutic approach (S-S).

The U-U process is the most primitive. It demands the least from the patient in terms of previous cognitive development or present cognitive ability. We differentiate between the two because, in terms of psychogenetic retardation, the previous level of cognitive development may not necessarily be representative of present functioning ability. We do not imply that this form of play therapy be used only with the most severely retarded. The level of measured intelligence is not important. Rather we are interested in the level of functional behavior. The child whose behavior indicates a lack of consciousness of self, who seems too impulsive, or who appears to be driven through what is described as "organic driveness" to act out feelings of hostility, destructiveness, or general aggressiveness, without seeming to have a basis for this behavior, or conversely is withdrawn and rejects the environment or major portions of it, seemingly without cognitive basis, is best served by a therapeutic process in which the structure has been, if not eliminated, at least modified to such an extent that it appears to the child as if there were no structure. Traditional play therapy methods may also be effective with this type of child but the structure provided or imposed by the materials in the traditional setting do not enable him to develop his imagination to the same extent. They do not enable him to invent activities which will provide an outlet for social interaction, nor do they enable him to express whatever portion of hyperactivity is due to "driveness" in a socially acceptable manner.

The importance of unstructured materials lies in the patient's greater ability to control, create, change, and develop play activity with them. He can learn that he is a person capable of creating and controlling materials. This paves the way for learning that he can control himself and eventually allows him to interact with others. He can learn that he is not necessarily a dangerously destructive person and he can see that his impulses have been primarily destructive to himself. He can learn that his ideas and efforts can produce tangible differences in reality, e.g. the change in the size or shape of a piece of clay is due to his behavior. The patient does not destroy unstructured materials, some may get used up, but such materials are thought of as being expendable and the concept of destruction does not enter into it. If he tears a piece of clay in two, he does not destroy it but simply has two pieces of clay which he can recombine. He may become aware of the fact that it was he who created the two pieces and in a psychological sense, produced new material from what existed previously.

The indications from U-U therapy and the therapist's tasks become clearer if we think of the specific goals. The therapist's tasks are based on fairly clear criteria for choosing between two major modes of responding to the patient. One mode is a positive response which is reinforcing. A second mode is a negative response which is blocking or intruding. The decision of when to respond in either way is based on the basic goals of this form of play therapy. These goals are threefold. The *first* goal is recognition of self. This refers to the child's gaining a sense of control over his environment, realizing the freedom to follow his own ideas and sensing that he is a real person. It is the primary goal because the child must be encouraged to develop motivation for growth and become able to deal with more challenging problems. The child with no awareness of self is completely unable to utilize any of the growth-producing elements of his environment.

The *second* goal involves gaining understanding that impulses can be controlled. This is a form of conditioning whereby the patient becomes aware that he is able to control sudden intense drives. These patients have been unable to direct their behavior in a socially acceptable manner in the past and this fact has given rise to frustration, guilt, and lack of self concept which has been partially responsible for the presence of the emotional disorder.

The *third* goal is training the child to live within social boundaries. These boundaries in an unstructured situation are slight, but they are reflective of greater limits which society imposes. This is a matter of learning to respond to the behavior of others in a controlled manner and learning to contribute a mutually conceived project in group situations. These children usually have been unable to work through their own problems with the resources they have available and so have not had sufficient psychic energy to participate with their peers or society. Thus, they tend to reject their peers, to fight with them when intruded upon, and generally behave in a way disruptive to any sort of activity.

The next of the four procedures is that which utilizes unstructured materials with a structured therapeutic approach (U-S). This method is not new to the therapeutic field and is found in the activities of the occupational therapist, music therapist, recreation therapist, and other similar workers. One of the differences is the relationship between the patient and the therapist. Where this relationship is close and warm, the therapist is able to play the role of a model. Where the relationship is not based on an interchange of feeling, but facilitates a setting where the patient feels safe to carry out his behaviors, this is usually described as special therapy but not given the title of psychotherapy.

We are not claiming psychotherapy for only the procedures which we have described, but rather state that the nature of these kinds of playroom activities tend to set up the interpersonal relationships between the therapist and the patient which is required for psychotherapy to take place. The important factor is the concept that the patient is able to translate his desires into socially acceptable behavior by learning to anticipate what would be acceptable to the therapist. This prejudgment comes both from what he has observed the therapist doing and what, based on previous experience and insight, he judged that the therapist expected him to do. The therapist functions as a representation of the more democentric aspects of society and becomes a model upon which the patient may test his behavior. It should be underlined that the end-product is not of great importance, but the general procedures followed by the patient in attempting to create a product are important. Thus, it does not matter how good a belt emerges from the leather, but it does matter that the patient is able to sufficiently control his behavior, his impulses, and his general acting out tendencies to make a belt. We can understand this if we remember the times a child will go out to play, will call it "going out to play" but will nonetheless get a hammer and some nails and start making something. He feels that while he is making these things he is playing. What is important is that the activity itself takes on significance because he feels he is producing a product, but the efforts to create the product serve the function of play in terms of building imagination, helping toward creativity, and improving understanding of the surrounding world.

The *first* goal of the U-S method is the development of an improved self-concept. We have already established recognition of self but this uniting of self-image with objective reality in terms of actual ability becomes a form of improving self-concept by giving self-confidence where it is lacking, or bringing it to the reality level where it seems to be distorted. This goal is important if the child is to be able to live in the community at his level. This type of child must have a self-concept that will be consistent with his ability but will not be so self-depreciating that he cannot function up to his potential. Rather it must permit him to recognize that there are many things he cannot do, but also that there are many things that he can do, and when this recognition has been established and accepted it can be said that the therapy has been successful.

The *second* goal for this type of therapy involves improved impulse control. A child who realizes that impulses can be controlled may find this knowledge a two-edged sword in that he may still have a problem in controlling his impulses; he knows that he can control them and thus may feel guilty and upset because he does not. We have a self-reinforcing process where the feelings of social uneasiness increase because the child is not doing something he knows he can do. Play therapy improves impulse control by increasing understanding that the basic desires can be satisfied in a socially acceptable manner. It is not the desires themselves that are at fault but rather his knowledge of what to do about them.

The *third* goal involves the improvement of ability to interact socially. The child having learned that there are limits in society, has to learn where the limits are imposed, how they are imposed, and the difference between major limits and minor limits. This is related to social reality. The first impression on learning there are limits is that it is as great a crime to walk on the grass as it is to steal a ball. Both are treated as equal sins, both are treated with equal daring if he decides to be hostile. Here the improvement of his ability to interact socially will help him learn to make the appropriate differentiations within the social requirements.

The third of the four procedures utilizes structured materials with a generally unstructured approach (S-U). The materials and approach, the indications for the psychotherapy, and the goals are all similar to traditional play therapy procedures.[2] We define this method as involving, as do the traditional precepts of play therapy, toys which have a preconceived construct as to their use, in a situation where the therapist has no preconception as to what he wants the child to play. The setting in the S-U situation is more narrowly conceived than in the usual play therapy room, the toys are often more narrowly conceived, but in general the method can be thought of as one primarily aimed at inviting thematic play and it is for this reason that we have described it in terms of the traditional precepts.

The goals of the S-U method are *first* to help the child build relationships with people at the level of understanding that a more democentric, more expressive interaction with his environment can be more gratifying than the egocentric, self-contained attitudes and behaviors which he has previously adopted. This is gained through the expression in play of the conflicts and hos-

tilities which he feels and through associations which the therapist helps provide concerning acceptable means of expressing
feelings without destroying the environment or the interpersonal
relationship.

The *second* goal is to help the child deal with social and cultural realities in terms of the fact that he is in a position to create
some joy and gratification in his environment, if he will learn to
deal with the reality of society and not constantly run contrary
to expectations and demands.

The *third* goal attempts to help the child evaluate his past
experiences in the light of new attitudes, to aid in his development and to establish personal goals in terms of a realistic level
of aspiration and a realistic consciousness of self. It may be ar-
gued that a child with little ability or potential is a preconceived
failure in this kind of therapy. However, if a child is at a sufficiently high functional level to be brought into the S-U type of therapy,
he has sufficient psychic energy and sufficient potentials to contribute socially at various levels and the understanding of these
levels will enhance his personality rather than increase the frustration.

The fourth procedure utilizes structured materials with a
structured therapeutic approach (S-S). This form is based on
the premise that many personality aberrations are due to the
child's being aware that he cannot function at a level equal to that
of his peers. This assumption does not require that the child have
a knowledge of all of the ramifications of the disturbance, but
rather an observation that he is not performing as well, in any
area, as his peers. Thus, if a child feels that if he could tell time
he could compete with his peers, the S-S type of therapy may very
specifically take time out to teach him how to tell time. Therapists would not necessarily agree with the child that this was the
source of his problem but having taught him how to tell time the
therapist would help the child understand that there were still
problems and that possibly the child could find better ways of
working them through in terms of his present potentials. This
may take one play session or it may take a number of sessions.
The therapist must maintain rapport and patient contact by participating in the activities so that the two of them are trying to

deal with the problem together, rather than the child finding himself isolated. At no time should the therapist set up a problem and then psychologically go away leaving the patient to work it out for himself. Rather they attempt to work it through together, permitting the patient to feel that he has an ally, though the final solutions must come from the patient and not the therapist. The three goals are the following: a) the improvement of the level of social maturity through the development of improved cognitive function; b) the development of understanding on the part of the child as to where he fits into his milieu; and c) the building of reality relationships leading to improved levels of aspiration.

The brief outline above has set up forms of play therapy which in effect are forms of behavior required for survival in the community. Society seems to structure itself around the retardate in terms of these U-U, U-S, S-U, and S-S situations. The less-structured aspects of community living daily present the individual with unstructured stimuli, e.g. rain and wind. In such an unstructured relationship to the community, particular demands are not placed upon him but he must, nonetheless, respond properly, e.g. getting out of the weather or wearing proper clothing. More structured situations present highly structured stimuli in structured relationship to the community such that the individual is not free to make a decision but instead must go along with the decisions society has already made, e.g. stoplights. If the child learns through his play to cope with these problems in a controlled manner, it becomes possible that he may also be able to carry this learning into daily living as an adolescent and as an adult. The major gains from play therapy are the ability to know the critical demands of the community and the ability to have had success experiences in dealing with these demands. This creates a personality pattern which is acceptable to the community so he can be permitted to remain and to contribute to the community.[10]

RECENT DEVELOPMENTS

The most important current questions to be considered in play therapy come under the broader heading of appropriate procedures for delivering services in community clinics and community areas. There are a limited number of trained psychotherapists available, and an unlimited number of potential clients who require the type of behavior modification or play therapy which we have described. As the clinic picture improves, as comprehensive community mental health and mental retardation programs expand to greater numbers of communities, the problem seems to get worse because improved case finding reveals increasing numbers of children who could benefit greatly by these services. The answer would seem to be in modifying three aspects of the approach: *first,* to take a harder look at the question of one-to-one type of therapeutic relationships; *second,* to reevaluate the necessary training of a qualified play therapist; and *third,* to reevaluate the role of parents and the family in the therapeutic milieu of the child.

The question of reexamining the one-to-one relationship in play therapy goes even deeper than the question of seeing a child alone or in a group. Is an intensive intervention required to modify the child's behavior, would a different type of intervention help, or is an intervention really called for? In looking at the question of case finding or the use of play in a diagnostic situation (Chap. 9),[7] one of the factors of which the therapist or mental health worker must be constantly aware is not how the child in question plays but how he plays in relationship to the other children with whom he must play. Modes of play and peer interaction which may be considered unacceptable in some areas of the community may be very acceptable in other areas, and it is part of the responsibility of a successful play therapy program to maintain the ability of the child to survive among his own peers and in his own community. Therefore, for the therapist to intrude with a model of behavior inconsistent with the child's personal model as found in his home, neighborhood, etc., would in the long run be destructive to the child even though it may modify certain behaviors.

The first question is whether the child successfully plays in a group in a manner consistent with the demands of his peers and his community. If he does, then regardless of what types of learning disabilities or school problems have emerged, play therapy as we have described it, may not be a treatment of choice. Rather than approach the child as though we were dealing with a pathological problem it is better to approach the behavior as an educational and cultural question, which may not even be posed as a problem but merely as a different way of behaving. We need to help the child and the surrounding community recognize that differences do exist, that they should be accepted as differences, and should not be labelled as pathologies.

If on the other hand, the child emerges from group diagnostic play sessions as not being able to interact with his peers, as having different or peculiar behavior modes in relationship to his peers, and becoming as rejected by them as by the more dominant community elements, then we feel that he has emerged as a psychotherapy candidate whose behaviors must be modified if he is to survive. One cannot automatically say that a child with a learning disability or a school problem also has a behavior disorder, just because his behavior is inconsistent with that experienced in other more comfortable sections of town.

The second question is a matter of knowing what play experiences are required for retarded children from poverty areas, from the ghetto, from the barrios, to permit them to function with children from the more comfortable areas so that a larger community of learning can be achieved. We need to talk about group play experiences similar to those in integrated schools. These are in a sense therapeutic, in that the interactions and experiences improve the coping strategies of the individual children involved, though they are not within themselves to be considered therapy in that there is no planned modification of behavior going forward. The community clinics or various types of community mental health and mental retardation services may have to provide some of this variety of play experiences if the community itself is not able to do so, and it may be necessary to open up recreation activities, sponsoring the use of gymnasiums, playgrounds, etc., for a large variety of play experiences which the communities, because of their tight geographical divisions, may not be able to provide. This will permit children who have come to the attention of these services because of learning disabilities and maladaptive behaviors, to profit from a variety of experiences but not necessarily having to be considered as candidates for intensive psychotherapy. This is a therapeutic experience, however, and one which is probably in many respects more important than psychotherapy in that it permits the child to change certain coping skills without having been specifically designated as a therapy patient and thus isolated from his peers.

It is to be expected that out of these supervised play experiences which we have described, there will emerge certain children whose maladaptive behavior is intolerable to their peers. These children will have a combination of learning disabilities including some evidence of retardation and a definite impairment in their adaptive behavior.[1] Typically, small play groups aimed at modifying similar behaviors can readily be formed. Two types of play therapy groups begin to feasibly evolve: one based on the convenience of the therapist where all of the children present have similar needs and it is a matter of dealing with these needs on a group basis rather than on an individual basis; the other where it is felt that certain types of peer interactions will speed up and support the therapy process through imitation and counter-imitation. In the first instance, a small group of three or four youngsters, all of whom have the same presenting difficulty, can be brought into a similar group procedure usually at the S-U or U-S level (these two forms being more readily adaptable to group procedures than either the U-U or S-S levels). The therapist, through developing both a pattern of mutual intrusion by utilizing the other children in the group as co-therapists around a single problem, and by setting up certain types of limits, may help the group achieve the necessary behavior modification.

The other alternative is based on the fact that it is valuable to mix groups of children with different coping modes (e.g. aggressive versus withdrawn or passive) because the children learn somewhat more readily from each other by imitating those behaviors which seem to be successful and rejecting those behaviors which seem to most usually cause punishment or intrusion.[9] However, in both these instances we end up with group therapy drawn from children who have been associated first in groups for diagnostic purposes and later in groups for richer and broader play experiences. This third level of group experience becomes a very highly specialized group approach which can come under the heading of "group therapy." It will ease the delivery of service problem by dealing with more children at one point than on a one-to-one basis, but it should be recognized that this reason is secondary to meeting the unique needs of the concerned children.

WHO DOES PLAY THERAPY?

If the types of group experiences we have described above are to be possible it is obvious that a greater number of play therapists have to be available. It is illogical to conceptualize at this time a vast increase in the number of doctoral level psychologists or other individuals doing play therapy at a highly professional level. In point of fact, the requirements for these individuals and the expansion of programs and services is such that most persons trained at this level are not giving direct service but rather find themselves in various administrative capacities where they are planning, organizing, and managing programs. We thus have the contradiction of the individual trained to provide the service not providing it, while at the same time the needs for such service are daily increasing. The answer is obviously not to take highly trained people out of the planning, administrative, and organizing roles, because the development of innovative programs and the total expansion of service, training, and research programs is dependent partly on that level of training and understanding. The answer would seem to lie in the other direction, i.e. beginning to train an increasingly large number of subprofessional personnel who can take on more and more responsibility in the service areas under the supervision of the more trained individual. Here one deals with a service-training paradigm which says that where there is an organized body of knowledge with a well-organized set of procedures and a low total impact from each specific decision, a relatively untrained person can perform. Where the knowledge and procedures are vague and where the impact of decision is extremely important (e.g. a decision to institutionalize a child) the services must be performed by a more highly trained or more competent individual.[11]

With this paradigm in mind it is very feasible to train a large number of subprofessional individuals to carry out the kinds of play therapy procedures which we have described. There is an organized body of knowledge with fairly well-organized procedures surrounding it and the individual decisions do not have a major long-range impact on the child. This would seem to be a ready-made situation for a subprofessionally trained individual who could step in under the supervision of a more highly trained person and carry out the actual play therapy processes. In point of fact, groups of such individuals who might be described as play therapy aides become even more effective and are able to provide a continuation of some of the requirements of one-to-one interaction while dealing with ever increasingly large groups of children who require this type of modification.

The important elements are first the relationship between the child and the therapists. This has to be a very warm, meaningful relationship and it is sometimes difficult to develop this kind of relationship with less trained individuals. With the above problem in mind we have set up a procedure which has been relatively successful. The senior therapist, typically the more thoroughly trained individual, sets up the therapy group. He may carry three, even four of the sessions, to insure that the patients have developed appropriate understanding of the therapeutic procedures, have fairly clear understanding of the limits and, in general, have begun to be part of a more concise and definite play therapy process, regardless of the method being used. At this point subprofessionally trained individuals are introduced into the therapy sessions and are maintained as co-therapists for an additional one or two sessions so that there may be several people in a therapy session (depending on the size of the patient group) with varying levels of background training. At the end of that period the senior therapist retires and the junior therapists then continue to maintain the sessions working together under the supervision of the senior therapist but now with full responsibility for the management of the cases and the establishment of the therapeutic procedures. It has been demonstrated that this type of transfer works very smoothly, that there is relatively little difficulty in making the transition, in fact less difficulty than under other circumstances because the group of patients do not develop the kind of fixed loyalty or transfer of affections which sometimes occurs in one-to-one relationships.

This type of procedure is also used as a teaching device for those learning psychotherapy. They can watch and discuss with the senior therapist the procedures from the beginning, even before they have been introduced as co-therapists and thus gain increased understanding before they come into actual charge of the case. If one of the co-therapists is to be specifically in charge it is also useful to introduce him from the beginning as a co-therapist so that any specific problems that may arise around building initial rapport can be handled as much by him as by the senior therapist. This gives the lesser trained therapist more confidence in his ability to deal with the problem.

If this procedure is to work efficiently one has to be primarily concerned with the levels of supervision. That is, the relationship between the co-therapists and the senior therapist becomes the key to success in this type of approach. One of the more effective ways of providing such supervision, taking into consideration time limitations, etc., is the establishment of teaching seminars whereby the supervision is provided not only by the senior therapist, leading such a seminar, but by all of the other participating co-therapists who would be discussing, questioning, and dealing with varying modes of approach. It would be possible for many different modes to emerge, all of which could be dealt with logically and consistently against the behavior of the child so that the most appropriate mode could be chosen. This type of supervision permits immediate review of the therapeutic interactions without having to absorb a great deal of the senior therapist's time in the one-to-one type of supervision. Here the old principle that the therapist in supervision is really himself a patient has to be lost in favor of a newer principle that the therapeutic person in modifying a child's behavior must use organized methods and reportable procedures. The specific emotional problems of the therapist, while important, cannot be permitted to dominate the supervisory sessions, or the search for procedures to be utilized with a given child will suffer. So that the supervisory sessions have to be based on the evolution of procedures and the logical understanding of why certain procedures work with some children and certain do not work, the main criteria being what works.

These subprofessional aides must be taught to use affect as one of their major devices for intrusion. All of the people participating in the therapeutic situation need an approach like silent screen actors. If the children do something unacceptable it must be made clear from the therapist's facial expression, from the words they use and other emotive behaviors, that this is not acceptable. Conversely, if the child does something of which they do approve, all of the participating therapists must light up, must react in one way or another indicating that they very highly approve of what the child is doing. This type of consistent reinforcement serves the group and individual process by immediately giving the child supportive or nonsupportive feedback for his behavior. It immediately tells other children where they may get supportive feedback and thus indicates what behaviors might be initiated or followed. It conversely tells what behaviors do not get supportive feedback and thus if they want rewards what behaviors need to be avoided. If the therapist follows the older mode of accepting the child's behavior without visible expression of acceptance or rejection the child will come to feel the therapist does not care, and that the behavior was not important. If the therapist does not care there is no particular reason why the child should care. If therapy procedures, particularly with less-professionally trained individuals, are to be effective, it must be immediately clear to the child when he is performing in an acceptable mode and when he is not.

Therefore, if the senior therapist can evolve a training program around a group of junior therapists who can follow specific concepts on a session-by-session basis, and who then receive intervening supervision to improve their understanding and if they can learn to transmit this to the child both through standard therapy procedures and through clearly expressive emotional responses, it is possible to reach a larger number of children with a larger number of personnel.

USE OF PARENTS AND HOME MILIEU

Another new development in modifying the manner in which services can be delivered to children is related to making greater use of the child's home milieu and incorporating parents or other adults into the therapeutic process. The therapy tradition with the mentally retarded has grown up in institutions where there was a solid, captive population. The better institutions maintained a therapeutic milieu in the sense that the aides in the cottages carried out certain procedures as directed and there was a broad pattern of continuity available. Typically, community services have not conceptualized doing psychotherapy with mentally retarded and this utilization of the full range of the child's milieu has not always been considered to be part of the procedure. However, falling back on the rule that the greater the degree of retardation the greater the need for a more directive type of therapeutic intervention, it becomes obvious that the period between sessions can be relatively destructive to the retarded child in that he will forget some of the experiences, will fall back into failure experiences and may, in general, retrogress.

This variation of time between sessions would seem to offer two alternatives, either see the child more often, which the busy schedules of clinics and other community services usually will not permit, or develop some sort of carry over into the child's home milieu. The second of these suggestions seems to be the most feasible and the processes are essentially a matter of working through with the parent, behavior modes whereby the child can move from maladaptive coping into more adaptive coping within the broad aspects of the home situation. This is a matter of working with the parents to determine what behaviors are most difficult for them, i.e. what aspects of the child's behavior they feel must be changed above all else. The parents can learn procedures which might permit changes through using behavior modification techniques, by being reinforcing about certain behaviors and intrusive or punishing about others. The child is given an opportunity for a broad pattern of continuity from what he has learned in play therapy on through to the home (though the parent does not necessarily do what the therapist does). Typically the parent does not have time with the requirements of housekeeping, a job, etc., to devote the kind of attention to all aspects of the child's behavior as is done in therapy. The parents *can* become aware each time the child carries out certain specific behaviors which are most annoying to them; they can have a procedure established to respond to that specific behavior so that at least in terms of the actions which are annoying them the most, they can carry out various interventions. In this way the child will learn to feel that their parents are interested in their behaviors and interested in their achievement of certain reward situations. Finally the parents can become rewarding individuals instead of the continuous punishing individuals that the parents of retarded children often tend to be.

One aspect of this as it relates directly to play therapy is the initiation of more directed play within the home situation. Here it is a matter of systematically teaching the child how to play and indicating what things he should be playing with and under what modes. This is not an attempt to limit his creativity by the parent coming and saying, "Okay, play with your trucks now," but rather a very systematic effort saying, "This is a truck," "It has four wheels," "They go around," and "You play with it in the following manner, here." The child may or may not wish to play with it at that time, and the parent should permit him to make his own choices, but at least an effort has been made to give him the opportunity to understand what playing with a truck implies. Quite often this is the instruction he has been lacking. It has been assumed he knew how to play with a truck. He may not play with it at the moment the parent discusses it, simply because children do not always do things at the moment their parents tell them to, but usually he will come back and play with it later when it can be his decision and the play activity will thus move forward. This feeling that he is doing something that his mother wants him to do, that she has shown him to do, and that other children around him do, adds to his repertoire of success experiences and he begins to achieve the same aspects of self-confidence and self-concept which become the elementary goals in the more intensive forms of play therapy. Thus parents can play a very clear-cut role without themselves having to be therapists.

Parents from the ghetto or low poverty areas of town should be trained to function as co-therapists or therapy aides within the clinic setting. If these kinds of community settings can be established within the geographical living space of the child, his own neighborhood, or adjacent neighborhoods of the inner-city, the barriers which interfere with his present learning, such as language differences[3] or other major divisions between the child's personal culture and the more dominant culture can become non-intervening variables in the play therapy situation. The therapist and the child will speak the same language, they will have come from similar cultural backgrounds and will have certain understandings between them before the child enters therapy. At that point it becomes much simpler for the specific behaviors which need to be modified to be considered. Thus, individuals from the same social cultural areas have to be trained as therapy aides. Further, there seems to be increasing supporting reasons that inclusion of the parents speeds up the therapy processes and is to the advantage of the total service program.[5]

As a final point in this area, it has to be recognized that children of different sexes play differently and that similar play therapy procedures cannot subsume a universality. On the other hand there is no particular reason to say that a boy should not play with dolls or that a girl should not play with a hammer. The sexual differences if anything need to be minimized in play therapy so that the children can learn to play and interact with each other while at the same time recognizing that there are sexual differences and that these are going to be important eventually for life adjustments. The sexual differences center around the child understanding his role in society but not around the kinds of toys or the things with which he plays. It is extremely important in dealing with the more disadvantaged child from poverty areas because it is likely that he has already been aware of sexual intercourse or physical interaction between sexes. The therapist cannot pretend that these do not exist nor can he pretend that this is the all-important aspect of play since in this child's milieu the heavy loadings of guilt which emerge in the more middle class areas are not present. Therefore these interactions have to be treated in the play situation as a normal everyday part of life along with the language that is associated with them. The therapist has to be totally accepting of this as part of the child's life while at the same time helping him realize that as a boy or girl, he or she has a certain and specific relationship to these events and that it is this relationship which must be worked through, understood, and around which appropriate coping strategies have to be developed.

CONCLUSION

In this chapter we have described some patterns which should emerge in attempting play therapy with the mentally retarded. We have pointed out that the main impetus of play therapy has to do with the function of structure within the child's environment, and the main function of the therapist becomes the manipulation of that structure in helping to modify the child's behavior. We have further pointed out that while play therapy is a regular and necessary part of the procedure of dealing with the emotionally disturbed, mentally retarded, or developmentally disabled child, that the kinds of procedures used must nonetheless take into consideration the level of disturbance or the level of retardation. We have suggested four particular kinds of procedures which have been successful in our experience.

Further we have underlined the need to develop a process of delivery of services to an increasingly large number of children while at the same time increasing the availability of manpower typically at the subprofessional or therapy aide level. We have underlined that the pathological model is not necessarily the best model for approaching the large number of disadvantaged, poverty children who behave differently than the more dominant community but who are not necessarily to be labelled as emotionally disturbed or "mentally ill." However, certain of these children will emerge as being atypical from their own peers and it is this atypical group of children who need therapeutic intervention. Finally, we have underlined the importance of including the parents or family in the therapeutic milieu of the atypical child so that the whole process can move forward at a more rapid and successful pace.

Since one aspect of adjustment has been the failure to recognize that situations exist which require coping, it is part of the function of play therapy first to point out the situations and then to help the patient learn to deal with them. This two-part procedure makes play therapy with the mentally retarded somewhat different than with higher mentalities where the major emphasis is on their learning to cope with situations with the basic assumption that they are already aware that the situations exist. This slight difference does require as we have indicated, different therapeutic approaches and different training for the clinical psychologists involved.[8] However, the results are rewarding both for the child and for the therapist and will carry us a long way towards improving the total mental health and learning potential of the children.

REFERENCES

1. American Association on Mental Deficiency: Manual on terminology and classification in mental retardation, 2nd ed. Monograph Supplement. *Am J Ment Defic*, 66, 1961.
2. Axline, Virginia M.: *Play Therapy*. Boston, Mass., Houghton Mifflin, 1947.
3. Baratz, Joan C.: Language and cognitive assessment of negro children. *J Am Speech Hearing Assoc*, 11(3):87-91, 1969.
4. Edmonson, Barbara, Leland, H., deJung, J. E., and Leach, Ethel M.: Increasing social cue interpretations (visual decoding) by retarded adolescents through training. *Am J Ment Defic*, 71(6): 1017-1024, 1967.
5. Hunt, J. McV.: Parent and Child Centers: Their Basis in the Behavioral and Educational Sciences. Presented 47th Annual Meeting, *American Orthopsychiatric Association*, San Francisco, March 25, 1970.
6. Leland, H., Nihira, K., Foster, R., and Shellhaas, M.: The Demonstration and Measurement of Adaptive Behavior. In Richards, B. W. (Ed.): *Proceedings of the First Congress of the International Association for the Scientific Study of Mental Deficiency*. Surrey, England, Michael Jackson Publishing Co., Ltd., 1968. 74-80.
7. Leland, H., and Smith, D. E.: *Play Therapy with Mentally Subnormal Children*. New York, Grune and Stratton, 1965.
8. Leland, H., Smith, D. E., and Barclay, A.: Report of the workshop on the training of clinical child psychologists in mental retardation. *Ment Retard*, 8(4):24-28, 1970.
9. Leland, H., Walter, J., and Toboada, A. N.: Group play therapy with a group of post-nursery male retardates. *Am J Ment Defic*, 63:848-851, 1959.
10. Shellhaas, M. and Nihira, K.: Factor analysis of reasons retardates are referred to an institution. *Am J Ment Defic*, 74(2):171-179, 1969.
11. Sutter, Emily, Leland, H., and Barclay, A. (Eds.): *Report of the Workshop on the Role of Subprofessionals in Clinical Child Psychology and Mental Retardation*, Sec. 1, Div. 12, A.P.A., 1200 Seventeenth Street, N.W., Washington, D.C., August 31, 1969.

Chapter 5

PSYCHOTHERAPY AND MENTAL RETARDATION

CHARLES M. MOODY

COUNSELING and psychotherapy of the mentally retarded and their families are not new areas of study. Many books and articles have been written about the subject. These publications reflect the assumption that the mentally retarded child and his family experience social and emotional stresses which can be alleviated by some form of psychotherapeutic intervention (or psychotherapy).

For the purposes of this chapter, the terms psychotherapy and counseling will be used interchangeably with the acknowledgment that this may be a departure from convention. Definitions of psychotherapy and counseling are known to be ambiguous. One author has prepared a consensus definition of psychotherapy as "effecting behavioral or personality changes in the direction of more effective adjustment through planned psychological, as opposed to medical, means."[4] Another defines counseling as "a form of interviewing in which the client is helped to understand himself more completely, in order that he may correct an environmental or adjustment difficulty."[14] Wiener[13] says if individuals are "primarily interested in getting advice on a concrete problem" then a counselor, rather than a psychotherapist, would be most appropriate.

Most psychological problems manifested in the retarded, and their families, will respond to therapeutic intervention only when the concentration on personality change (psychotherapy) is joined with an emphasis on resolving interpersonal and environmental difficulties through the use of collateral agents (counseling).

In general these two aspects of the therapeutic process have not been linked by many psychotherapists and others working in the mental health field. This may explain the tendency of many traditional agencies to avoid problems relating to retardation, whether they be in the family or the retarded person himself. In most instances the need for psychotherapy is acknowledged, but the family or individual is referred to a "specialized" facility, frequently physically or socially removed from the problem-solving arena, with the rationale that greater expertise will be available there.

There are some explanations for these actions. Many mental health professionals have had no more contact with the retarded than have the general public, and consequently find them strange and unmanageable and try to avoid them as clients. Professionals frequently share societal stereotypes regarding the retarded. For example, the belief that retardation is basically a static condition is sometimes enlarged to the assumption that pathological behavior in a retarded person is likewise static and hence not amenable to psychotherapeutic efforts.

Perhaps most damaging to the retarded and their families seeking help is the difficulty which many mental health professionals experience in trying to integrate other supportive services such as foster care, day treatment, etc. into the treatment plan. Though these criticisms are generally focussed on the broad mental health field, even specialized mental retardation facilities have shortcomings. Clinics which make extensive diagnoses and perform only minimal treatment, follow-up, and implementation of findings are examples of failure to meet the client's needs.

GENERAL OBSERVATIONS ON COUNSELING IN RETARDATION

Excessive Reliance on "Acceptance"

Olshansky[9] in his work on chronic sorrow, illuminated the tenacity with which some mental health professionals pursue parents of the mentally retarded to get them to "accept" the reality of their child's retardation. Ambivalent feelings toward a retarded child are often viewed as "the tip of the iceberg of acceptance" and are ferreted out and analyzed. The concept of "acceptance," and the common tendency to make it the basic goal of therapy, is largely a creation of professional myth-makers and, as a psychological abstraction, is decidedly unhelpful. To focus all therapeutic effort on the ambivalence of the parent toward the retarded child may not only be a fruitless task but may also neglect the other problems awaiting solution.

Professionals might ask themselves if parents are *denying* the fact that their child is retarded, not whether they are *accepting* this fact. And when ambivalence toward the child is present, it should be evaluated in terms of its impact, if any, on the child. Infrequent erratic emotional responses on the part of parents and even periodic regressions do not have to be negative factors. Even occasional withdrawal from the demanding life with a retarded child may be an indication of the parent's strength.

Need for Functional Assessments

Mental health workers counseling parents of the retarded need to develop a functional or performance assessment to complement the traditional psychopathological model. If parents of a retarded child, or a retarded adult for that matter, are able to mobilize themselves on behalf of their dependent child, then their functional response should generally be deemed adequate. If they are not able to mobilize themselves on behalf of the child, then their functional assessment is not adequate and intensive intervention is indicated. The presence of many clearly defined defense mechanisms is not, by themselves, serious signs if the family is functioning adequately and dealing with its responsibilities to the retarded child. If parents follow through on referrals, keep their medical appointments, come in for counseling and so forth, then, in spite of reaction formation, rejection, overprotection, ambivalence, denial, or any other defense mechanism, their performance must be viewed as adequate. Likewise, families who will not follow through on referrals, even when the usual psychopathological signs are absent, should be suspected of having underlying difficulties preventing them from appropriately managing their retarded child.

This plea for a functional evaluation is not a denial that serious psychopathology sometimes is present in the retarded person and his family. Indeed, pathology may be present and when this is clearly the situation, the person or family should receive prompt and appropriate attention.

Creative Use of Psychodynamic Knowledge

Psychotherapy with the mentally retarded and their families frequently requires a particularly creative use of one's psychodynamic knowledge. Combining the functional assessment with the traditional psychopathological model is necessary to gain an accurate understanding of the dynamics of behavior, *but* it is not always helpful to interpret these dynamics to the client. This is especially true when the demands of the retarded child in a family frequently require accommodation and adjustment rather than resolution. Defense mechanisms, even those which in a family without a retarded child might be viewed as neurotic, frequently facilitate this accommodation.

> A mother of a two-year-old retarded son requested diagnosis and counseling. This boy was the youngest of five children, the rest of whom were apparently normal and well-adjusted. Following counseling suggestions, the mother secured a place for him in a nursery program, joined other parents in a counseling group and followed a medical regime designed to minimize his physical difficulties. Though his retardation was severe she verbalized expectations which were clearly unrealistic including the wish that he would someday marry and be self-supporting. The mother's functioning was viewed as appropriate and was meeting her child's needs. Her unrealistic verbalizations were not challenged and in no way seemed to interfere with other family members or the child's behavior or adjustment.

Many times counselors and therapists are required to absorb feelings, frequently hostile, which have been collecting within a family for some time. It is important that these feelings be accepted and understood and that the therapist not succumb to the temptation to retaliate or to point out the mechanism of projection and/or displacement which may seem so clearly present. By expressing himself, the client usually resolves the issue sufficiently to move ahead, which is, after all, a primary purpose of treatment.

Families who verbally deny the retardation of their child can present unique treatment problems. The therapist will avoid many difficulties by not entering into an argument over the presence or absence of retardation or the degree to which it is or is not present. Instead, the quiet acceptance of these denials and the focussing upon programming and intervention are much more suitable and usually will be positively received.

> A young couple reluctantly sought help with their three-year-old boy who had been diagnosed as mentally retarded. The mother was particularly vigorous in her rejection of the diagnosis and in fact insisted the child was gifted rather than retarded. However, she agreed to placing him in a daily development program for retarded children (though continuing to insist he was not retarded) and also joined a parent counseling group. Over a period of two years her denial gradually lessened and she became active in community retardation activities. At no time was she "confronted" with the reality of the child's condition or was her behavior interpreted to her. The counseling assessment was that her actions (rather than words) were appropriate for the child's needs.

In the same vein, it is suggested that families be allowed to use euphemisms if they wish to. If a person is more comfortable with the term "slow learner," the word "retarded" should not be forced on them. Similarly, if they find solace in such words as "handicapped," "brain damaged," or whatever, this should be allowed as an apparent comfort to them and should not be identified as a symbol of their problems of "accepting" their child.

Finally, it is recommended that underlying problems within parents or other family members, which do not seem to be related to the retarded individual and do not seem to be affecting his functioning, be approached very obliquely, if at all. Families who seek assistance because of difficulties with their retarded child may not be receptive to intervention in other problems. To pursue these, in the face of family resistance, may jeopardize the relationship and not only destroy the opportunity to deal with the secondary problem, but also might remove the family from treatment, thereby losing the chance to work with the presenting problem of mental retardation.

> A middle-aged mother applied for counseling at a community mental health agency. Her moderately retarded fourteen-year-old son had been exhibiting aggressive physical behavior at school and at home. The school authorities had suggested she seek counseling.

Complicating and perhaps contributing to the boy's behavior was his parents' stormy marriage and his father's physical incapacity. The therapist focussed on the marital conflicts and the mother ceased treatment after three visits because this was not the problem as she viewed it. When she requested help from a specialized retardation agency the presenting problem was the same. Here the initial focus was on the boy and his problems. After only a few visits she was discussing her marriage and her husband's problems with no apparent hesitation. The boy's behavior improved and she seemed to gain a different perspective on her own situation. The first agency's focus on an underlying problem was enough of a threat that the mother fled from treatment, whereas in the second agency the emphasis was on the presenting problem and thus at an acceptable level to the client.

Of course when families are receptive to therapy focussed on underlying problems this should not be discouraged. Treatment of any problem affecting family functioning represents the ideal goal of therapy but for those unable to achieve the optimum, meaningful and helpful treatment should also be available at a level that can be accepted.

THE TREATMENT APPROACH

When Is Therapy Indicated?

Determining when psychotherapy is indicated is not an easy matter. There are guidelines which are of assistance, but the final decision frequently depends upon the skill, perception, and sometimes the intuition of the therapist as well as the client's wish to change. Even if treatment seems clearly indicated, a problem frequently exists in convincing the individual or family that this is so. The point at which a receptive response to the treatment suggestion will be received is difficult to identify and depends on a variety of factors including motivation, interest, and accessibility, among others.

The Family

Counseling with families of the retarded is generally indicated when the parents are having difficulty making realistic plans for their child or are unable to mobilize themselves on behalf of the child once the plans are made. As stated earlier, verbalizations which have pathological qualities are not sufficient to indicate the need for treatment unless they are accompanied by overt action, or lack of action, which directly affects the child. However, when parents are unable, or refuse, to take advantage of opportunities for education or other services for their child, therapeutic intervention is strongly indicated.

When family stability or family relationships are affected, counseling is also usually indicated. Determining when this is taking place presents other difficulties, but when an apparently stable marriage is beginning to show stress, or when siblings of the retarded child are beginning to manifest signs of maladaptive behavior, one could assume that the family stability is in danger and intervention would be indicated.

Counseling may also be appropriate when a family is undergoing a crisis of any sort, directly related to the retarded member, or only indirectly affecting him. The dependency of the retarded person frequently thrusts him into prominent consideration in issues which would only be of peripheral concern if he were not retarded. The impact of these issues can frequently be eased by timely therapeutic involvement.

The Individual

When counseling is being considered for a retarded person, a flexible approach is necessary. Age differences and intellectual and functional variations require careful assessment. A technique that is useful with a mildly retarded adolescent might be inappropriate for a severely retarded youngster or any young child regardless of intellectual ability.

Generally, therapy can be of assistance if a person's achievement, at any level, is hampered by emotional problems. With children the therapeutic goal could be to alleviate emotional symptoms so that learning patterns would improve and behavior become more adaptive and less inappropriate. With retarded adolescents and adults therapy can minimize behavioral problems or other factors which might be preventing an individual from maximum functioning in a work training activity or socialization program, or which might be contributing to maladaptive behavior in the home.

Beck[2] has said that psychotherapy should be aimed at increasing the comfort of all people concerned with a trying situation. Professionals can do a number of things to help achieve this goal among the retarded:

Identify and deal with crises as they arise.

Establish "open door policies" which result in services that are useful and utilized by families and the retarded person.

Continue to search for techniques and methods which help relieve the stress and increase the comfort of persons affected by the problems of mental retardation.

Counseling as Part of the Diagnostic Process

Parents of retarded children are under exceptional stress when their child's condition is being evaluated. The demands placed upon the counselor at this time are likewise unique and require particular sensitivity. Counseling at this period can only be effective to the extent that the basic diagnostic process is thorough and accurate. The parent's primary concern is usually directly connected with the child's impairment and what this portends for the future. Counseling can be most successful if the therapist recognizes this and capitalizes on it as much as possible. The parents will frequently ask questions and these should be dealt with directly and not be viewed as neurotic symptoms or as an inability to grasp the magnitude of what is facing them. Questions regarding the causes of the retardation, the chances of it recurring in subsequent children, and the prognosis for the child should be discussed and parents should be told directly when answers are not available.

Parental feelings of anger or outrage (or similar emotions) are frequently seen during diagnostic interviews and should be understood and accepted rather than countered. The temptation to help the parents "work through" their feelings should be curbed, since it is questionable if this goal is achievable at this time. The therapeutic approach should be empathic and supportive. An insensitive or aggressive approach at this point may drive the family out of treatment.

Sometimes families show little open reaction, if any at all, to a diagnostic revelation of retardation. When the therapist is convinced that profound feelings are present, though as yet un-spoken, these should be approached cautiously until a strong re-lationship is established. Again the danger lies in a treatment ap-proach that is too threatening and might result in the family flee-ing from counseling.

Interpreting diagnostic findings is best handled over a pro-longed period of time. The enormity of what the parents are being told, even when it confirms what they have suspected for some time, is frequently sufficient to prevent them from absorb-ing more than just a little information at a time. The efforts of the most skilled therapist can be blocked by this situation. Stretching out the diagnostic interpretation can minimize the tendency of some parents to seek other experts in the next clinic in the hope the conclusions will be different, and can provide much greater opportunity for questions to be asked, answered, and understood than can one or two sessions.

Psychotherapy with Parents of Retarded Infants or Small Children

There are several issues to be examined before counseling is attempted with parents of retarded children. Medical diagnosis of the child must be underway or completed. The therapist and the parents must be satisfied that the evaluation is thorough. And the parents must be showing signs of accommodating to the diagnostic implications. If their resistance to the diagnosis is pro-longed, further counseling will be of questionable value until the resistance is resolved.

Glasser, in his writings on Reality Therapy,[6] stresses the im-portance of the client's plan in the treatment relationship. I be-lieve this concept has particular application for therapists work-ing with parents of retarded children. Many parents find it easier and more productive to begin making specific plans for their re-tarded child than to examine their feelings about the child. Those parents who find difficulty mobilizing themselves can usually be stimulated and helped to reach the point of initial planning.

The process of planning can accomplish several tasks. It de-mands that the parents look beyond themselves for resources and opportunities for their child and view these resources realistically in terms of their child's needs. The process can require them to face directly some of their ambivalence about the child and to recognize that even retarded children have some abilities and potentials to balance their liabilities. Planning frequently rekindles the individual's basic optimism which may have been dimmed by the birth of a retarded child and the broad tendency in our society, a tendency shared by some professionals, to view this as a calamity beyond comparison.

Placement

The question of whether a child should remain in his own home or be placed in an alternative living situation frequently arises in counseling and many times is the basis for the referral in the first place. In the past the question of placement was one that frequently polarized professionals and confused parents seeking assistance with this dilemma. Some therapists insisted placement should never be encouraged while others felt that children falling in certain diagnostic categories should always be placed.

Placement is indeed a realistic plan for some families and an unrealistic one for others. In helping parents determine whether placement is appropriate the therapist must assess the strengths of the community, the presence and attitudes of siblings and above all, the desires and wishes of the parents.

The therapist should strive to maintain the counseling relationship in such a way as to allow the parents to make a balanced decision regarding placement. Attempts should be made to help parents avoid an early "commitment to placement" particularly when this does not seem feasible in view of the community's resources. Some parents request counseling after having been advised by a family physician or other influential professional to place their retarded child. After much anguish they have accepted this recommendation and then are stunned to learn of waiting lists, priority admissions, and the other harsh realities which mental retardation professionals deal with daily.

Collateral Services

Traditional counseling and psychotherapy concentrate primarily on the interchange between patient and therapist and only secondarily on collateral services. Collateral services, however, can be one of the greatest assets a counselor can offer parents of a retarded child if these are integrated with a focus on the parent's feelings, attitudes, and conflicts toward the child. As suggested earlier, some therapists may not be comfortable in the use of outside resources but the amelioration of unproductive or conflicting feelings within parents and other family members may hinge on the extent to which community services are involved.

In the treatment context the therapist should be willing to discuss specific problems within the home which are related to the child's adjustment and development. These might require discussions of feeding problems, toilet training, behavioral management, and other such concerns which might not normally be considered part of the therapist's skill repertoire. For example, a referral to a specialist in behavior modification technique could be one of the most helpful services a counselor could offer a family who is being severely tried by behavioral problems which are not responding to more traditional methods of intervention.

Techniques

Recommendations on the use of specific therapeutic techniques to be used with parents of retarded children are difficult to make. Techniques depend upon the training of the therapist, his philosophical and theoretical orientation, and above all, his skill.

Some general comments, however, might be of some value. Treatment interviews with one rather than both parents should be approached with caution and the pitfalls noted. Sometimes individual interviews cannot be avoided and certainly they are better than no interview. However, conjoint interviews have several distinct advantages.[11] Perhaps most outstanding is the fact that both parents are involved in the examination, and hopefully, the resolution of their problem and, thereby, they develop or enhance mutual responsibility for their child. Dependency relationships between husband and wife can be minimized and interdependence fostered. Distortions of the therapist's role are lessened. One parent will find it more difficult to project responsibility onto the other for the retardation or problems resulting from it.

A woman requested counseling because of concern for her retarded daughter. She was very reluctant to involve her husband but agreed to the therapist's insistence that he come if at all possible.

She phoned between interviews and expressed her fear that the child's retardation was hereditary through her husband's family but could not bring this up in the treatment sessions. The medical diagnosis was such that it ruled out hereditary factors and eventually the wife was able to come to grips with her projection and deal more appropriately with her child and her husband. She allowed him to assume more responsibility for the child and to assist in the girl's care. It is doubtful if this sharing of responsibility could have been attained if the mother had been seen alone.

When older, nonretarded siblings are present in the family it is advisable to involve them in the family counseling. Frequently they play a key role in the family's ability to deal effectively with the problems presented by the presence of a retarded child.

Once families have worked through acute crises and are carrying out an effective plan for their child, then it is suggested they be put into a "maintenance therapy" program. These programs can take various forms and are somewhat dependent upon the interests and needs of the family and the resources in the community.

If children are in school or in another program, maintenance therapy can be a closely integrated component of the program. Group counseling would be the most common technique and the goals would be to sustain an adequate functioning level, provide parents with the opportunities to share experiences, draw strength from one another and gain comfort in the knowledge that others are facing and dealing successfully with the problems of retardation.

A variation in the group approach is to use time-limited groups. These groups would meet a specified number of times, generally between six and ten sessions. Some parents seem to prefer this form of group treatment and will contract and follow-through with it, whereas they are reluctant to involve themselves in open-ended group therapy.

Psychotherapy with Parents of Retarded Adolescents or Adults

The goals of counseling with parents of retarded adolescents or retarded adults differ from those sought with parents of younger children. By the time a retarded child reaches adolescence or adulthood, the parents have made a basic accommodation to his handicap. In many cases this accommodation has been satisfactory for the parents and the child, in others it has not. Yet, good or bad, the parents' adaptation to life with a retarded person is the product of many years of experience and this life style will be resistive to change. The counselor can most productively use his skills and the therapeutic time if this is taken into consideration.

Parents of retarded adolescents usually seek counseling assistance because of specific problems with the youngster. Frequently there is a crisis. Typically these crises revolve around aggressive behavioral reactions, threatened or actual sexual acting out and other problems which are paralleled in many nonretarded teenagers and young adults.

> A divorced mother requested crisis counseling for herself and her fifteen-year-old moderately retarded daughter. This child was the oldest of seven children and had been sexually abused by a number of neighborhood boys and men for several months. The mother feared the daughter would become pregnant or be physically injured or worse and felt her best efforts to supervise the child were insufficient. Counseling focussed on alternatives to home care and a decision to place the child in a foster home was made based on the needs of the child and the mother.

When parents present problems such as outlined above, their anxieties are very high, and rightfully so, and immediate intervention is required. Sometimes supportive counseling and allowing parents to ventilate their feelings will be sufficient. However, other times the intervention must include the use of collateral services if the crisis is to be overcome.

When the retarded child reaches adolescence, parents will sometimes request counseling with the onset of puberty itself being the crisis. Sexual drives are awakening, the gaps between physical development and psychological and intellectual capacity become even more pronounced and there is a new concern for the future.

The "chronic sorrow" as described by Olshansky[9] now becomes clearly pronounced. Many times there are no answers to the questions posed by parents because, as Olshansky suggests, the problems lie within the mother and father and not the child. In other instances the therapist can help the parents reach a workable equilibrium by offering a variety of services: arranging for guardianship, foster home or institutional care, referral to activity centers or workshops, helping locate respite care, and so forth.

Most parents of the retarded have great strength and resiliency. This is illustrated by parents who continue on indefinitely with courage, cheerfulness, and patience as they cope with the constant challenge without yielding to the burden. This coping behavior can be encouraged and supported if competent and yet sympathetic help is available when the stresses threaten to become overwhelming.

Psychotherapy with the Retarded

One of the first matters to be considered in counseling the retarded is the degree of intellectual deficit that is present. There is little doubt that counseling with the retarded can be of great value though it becomes increasingly challenging with an increasing degree of retardation. There is a point when the amount of counseling effort is no longer warranted though this point varies from person to person.

The Retarded Child

Therapists considering the use of psychotherapeutic techniques with young retarded children must ask themselves the same questions they would ask when considering treatment for any young child. One concern is whether the investment of time is justified by the potential return. In most cases, it is far better to concentrate one's therapeutic efforts on the parents. Their constant involvement with their child puts them in a better position to modify or restructure behavior than can be achieved through an occasional treatment hour. Sometimes treatment goals cannot be attained by counseling solely with the parents. In that case, work with the child and/or the family is justified.

A second question to be resolved before treatment ensues is whether psychotherapy, either with child or parents, is preferable or should situational stresses be investigated. For example, if behavioral problems in a seven-year-old are related to pressure or frustration in school they will not respond to treatment unless the pressure at school is lessened. A child's aggressive behavior toward peers might respond more readily to a prescription for socialization than a futile course of counseling.

Techniques used with retarded children differ little from those used with the nonretarded. Play therapy is a favorite technique with many therapists and is particularly applicable and helpful for nonverbal children. Therapeutic play activities in small groups are sometimes used either alone or in conjunction with individual treatment. Group therapy is quite effective after the child reaches puberty and is widely used with the mildly retarded of all ages.

The Adolescent and Adult

Many retarded teen-agers and adults can be helped by psychotherapeutic means to unravel problems and conflicts blocking them from utilizing their full potential or achieving at a realistic level of satisfaction. Professionals using these methods with the retarded have had enough successful experience to convince them that many counseling approaches have merit.

In general, psychotherapy should be considered if the retarded person is manifesting emotional or behavioral symptoms which are interfering with his adjustment or his ability to utilize his intellectual, social, or vocational potential. This prescription for treatment is similar to that used with the nonretarded and techniques vary only slightly. Therapists working with the retarded usually avoid focussing on insights and using reflective therapy and frequently take an active role in the therapeutic interaction. Transference phenomena and behavioral dynamics are noted and may well influence the direction of treatment, but they are rarely interpreted to the client.

> A moderately retarded woman in her early twenties was referred for treatment by her mother with whom she lived along with several younger siblings. The mother's complaint was her daughter's extreme profanity and hostility toward her 16-year-old brother. The daughter had limited verbal skills but told how her brother provoked her, but in a manner not seen by the mother. Counseling focussed on helping the daughter to tolerate some of the provocations, to modify her response to them (i.e. substitute more appropriate language for the

profanity) and to recognize that mother would punish her for her behavior regardless of the circumstances. This approach, along with general supportive counseling, resolved the presenting problem and seemed to significantly alter the family interaction patterns and contribute to a general lessening of tension within the family.

The primary treatment focus generally involves a directive, structured approach. Acceptable treatment goals would be to help the individual identify elements within his life that are sources of conflict and help him find methods of resolving, minimizing, or avoiding these conflicts. While these goals are also sought in work with the nonretarded, most counselors specializing with the retarded play an aggressive and directive role in helping the person identify conflicts rather than depending on insight development.

Group methods are widely used with older retarded individuals and have many advantages. One of these is the opportunity to use two treatment methods or techniques at the same time. For instance members of a hobby or craft group can easily discuss their broader concerns in conjunction with or following their craft activities. The principles of group therapy methods and techniques apply in mentally retarded groups as they do anywhere else. The retarded can profit from one another's experiences just as normal people can, and they can learn and modify social skills through the group process. Those with limited verbal skills many times thrive in group counseling with more verbal fellow-group members, whereas they might be uncomfortable and nonproductive in individual counseling.

> Group therapy is an integral part of a sheltered workshop program for the retarded. Each workshop client is in two groups weekly. The therapy goals are to discuss, and hopefully resolve, individual and group problems affecting placement potential. The group has had excellent success identifying and curbing unrealistically high goals and in halting tendencies to scapegoat others for past failures. In one session a young man was blaming his recent job failure on personal differences with his employer. Group members reminded him of his previous statements about the positive relationship between them and he was able to concede that the job loss was due to his own shortcomings. In the same session a female client's inappropriate dress was challenged by group members. Though the group agreed she had the right to dress as she wished (her main

---

====

defense) they also clearly stressed that a continuation of this behavior would probably result in no job referral.

CONCLUSION

Counseling and psychotherapy are important tools in working with the mentally retarded. However, they must be used jointly with other techniques and services if we are to achieve our objectives of helping the retarded person and his family.

In this chapter I have emphasized three main areas of focus which I consider of major importance for professionals working in the field of mental retardation. Foremost is the critical need to utilize collateral services along with the interpersonal focus of the counseling process. Second is the importance of using a functional or performance assessment in work with the family of a retarded child. The third is an admonition to professionals, when developing treatment plans, to identify family and individual strengths and appropriate adaptive behavior thus avoiding the temptation to base treatment on "acceptance" or similar inexact psychological terminology.

If we apply our skills with creativeness, exercise our judgments with compassion and forethought, and view our retarded clients and their families as individuals with unique desires, ambition, and problems, our therapeutic efforts will prove rewarding to us, but above all will free the retarded person to live to his fullest potential as a member of the community.

REFERENCES

1. Beck, Helen L.: Casework with parents of mentally retarded children. Am J Orthopsychol, 32:870-877, 1962.
2. Beck, Helen L.: Counseling parents of retarded children. Children, 6:67-72, 1959.
3. Beck, Helen L.: The advantages of a multipurpose clinic for the mentally retarded. Am J Ment Defic, 66:789-794, 1962.
4. Bialer, Irv.: Psychotherapy and other adjustment techniques with the mentally retarded. In Baumeister, Alfred A. (Ed.): Mental Retardation: Appraisal, Education, Rehabilitation. Chicago, Ill., Aldine, 1967, pp. 139-180.
5. Cowen, E. L. and Trippe, M. J.: Psychotherapy and play techniques with the exceptional child and youth. In Cruickshank, W. M. (Ed.): Psychology of Exceptional Children and Youth. 2nd ed. Englewood Cliffs, N.J., Prentice-Hall, 1963, pp. 526-591.

6. Glasser, William: *Reality Therapy: A New Approach to Psychiatry.* New York, Harper and Row, 1965.
7. Gregg, Grace S.: Comprehensive professional help for the retarded child and his family. *Hosp Community Psychiatry,* 19:122-124, 1968.
8. Humes, Charles W., *et al.*: A school study of group counseling with educable retarded adolescents. *Am J Ment Defic,* 74:191-195, 1969.
9. Olshansky, Simon: Chronic sorrow: A response to having a mentally defective child. *Soc Casework,* 43:190-193, 1962.
10. Philips, Irving, *et al.*: The application of psychiatric clinic services for the retarded child and his family. In Szurek, S. A. and Berlin, I. N. (Eds.): *Psychosomatic Disorders and Mental Retardation in Children.* Palo Alto, Calif., Science and Behavior Books, 1968, pp. 166-180.
11. Schild, Sylvia: Counseling with parents of retarded children living at home. *Social Work,* 19:86-91, 1964.
12. Szurek, Stanislaus A. and Philips, Irving: Mental retardation and psychotherapy. In Philips, Irving (Ed.): *Prevention and Treatment of Mental Retardation.* New York, Basic Books, Inc., 1966, pp. 221-246.
13. Wiener, Daniel N.: *A Practical Guide to Psychotherapy.* New York, Harper and Row, 1968.
14. Wolberg, Lewis R.: *The Technique of Psychotherapy.* New York, Grune and Stratton, 1954.
15. Wortis, Joseph: Towards the establishment of special clinics for retarded children: Experiences and suggestions. *Am J Ment Defic,* 58:472-480, 1954.

Chapter 6

PRIMITIVE, ATYPICAL, AND
ABNORMAL BEHAVIORS

Frank J. Menolascino

INTRODUCTION

THROUGHOUT the United States, residential institutions for the mentally retarded are undergoing rapid change, accelerated by the establishment of community based facilities and programs for mentally retarded citizens. Indeed, one common reason for requesting admission to such a residential institution is the individual's inability to adjust to therapies within the primary community. Many of these community rejects frequently display an overlay of emotional disturbance which accounts for their adjustment problems. Accordingly, institutions for the retarded face the challenge of isolating and understanding the inner needs of these retardates so that they can benefit from available institutional programs and strive toward the goal of returning to the primary community.

In this chapter the author will review the three types of emotionally disturbed retarded individuals which he most frequently encountered as a psychiatric consultant to institutions for the mentally retarded. These three types are as follows: a) primitive behaviors, b) atypical behaviors, and c) abnormal behaviors. Each presents unique diagnostic, treatment-management and administrative problems which will be used to review and propose specific guidelines to better serve our mentally retarded fellow citizens.

PRIMITIVE BEHAVIOR

Primitive behavior usually is manifested by severely or profoundly retarded individuals who also display gross delay in psychosocial behavioral repertoires. Typically they are children

84

below the chronological age of eight years, and most commonly they are ambulatory. Primitive behaviors include very rudimentary utilization of special sensory modalities with particular reference to touch, position sense, oral explorative activity and essentially no externally directed verbalization. In the diagnostic interview, one notes much mouthing and licking of toys, excessive tactile stimulation such as "autistic hand movements" which are executed near the eyes, as well as skin-picking and body-rocking. The overall impression drawn from the observed behavior strongly suggests marked developmental delay of personality with organic fixation at a primitive behavior elaboration level. (Keep in mind the fact that such observation generally takes place against a backdrop of decreased animate and inanimate stimulation, usually within the bleak atmosphere of an institutional ward setting.)

From a diagnostic viewpoint, the very primitiveness of the child's overall behavior in conjunction with much stereotyping of same initially may suggest a psychotic disorder of childhood. However, these children do make eye contact and they will interact with the examiner quite readily despite their very minimal behavior repertoire. One might form the initial impression that both the level of observed primitive behavior and its persistency is secondary to intrinsically and extrinsically caused deprivation factors, though, at the same time, these children appear to have developmental arrest which is of primary or congenital origin. It should be noted that these children never possessed a functional ego at the appropriate chronological age, and they have little or no concept of self. Indeed, in many children with primitive behavior and profound mental retardation, one notes that there is an amorphic personality, or in other words, no functional personality structure.

The following case history illustrates the diagnostic-treatment challenges presented by this primitive behavior type.

> A six-and-one-half-year-old boy was seen for psychiatric consultation at the request of the ward team (i.e. a developmental specialist, social worker, physician, and psychologist) for diagnostic clarification and treatment recommendations. The youngster had been admitted for observation at the request of both his parents and the staff of the previous treatment setting whose transfer impression was, "Functions at the severely retarded level, but physically he looks so nor-

mal. He is not a very warm child. We wonder if he isn't an autistic child."

The personal history revealed that he was the third child in the family, born after an uneventful pregnancy to a twenty-six-year-old mother who had no prior history of obstetrical complications. Family history was negative for hereditary or degenerative diseases. His birth weight and clinical status in the early neonatal period were all within normal limits. By the age of six months, the child was described as passive, early developmental milestones were markedly delayed, and he displayed muscular hypotonicity. By the end of the first year of life, his developmental attainments were those of a four-month-old child, and he had undergone a variety of medical evaluations. No definite diagnostic impressions were obtained, and the parents were counseled to provide general stimulation for their youngster. Since this family placed a high premium on child care, they were not satisfied with such nonspecific diagnostic and management recommendations. Accordingly, between the ages of twelve months and forty-eight months, the boy underwent six more evaluations in different parts of our country, as well as three treatment programs (among which were Doman-Delacato and a speech therapy residential center). By the age of five years, this child was noted to be functioning at the twelve to sixteen month developmental level on formal psychometric assessment; his family was perplexed and was still shopping for diagnostic-treatment recommendation which would, "Really help him to grow like he should." (Mother's statement.) Medical reevaluation at age six was followed by parental rejection of the diagnostic impression of severe mental retardation, and the lad was entered into a course of megavitamin therapy. At the conclusion of this treatment, the boy was admitted to an institution for the retarded for further diagnosis, observation, and possible treatment. As previously noted, the admitting diagnosis was "possible autism."

Psychiatric examination of this rather handsome youngster revealed no physical signs or symptoms of delayed development except in finer hand movements, dull and vacant eyes, and no language present. He occupied himself continuously with quick hand movements approximately twelve inches from his eyes; he picked at a spot on his left wrist periodically; and initially he was only passively compliant with the examiner. However, on minimal inducement he interacted with the examiner by eye contact, patty cake and rolling a ball back and forth. The previously noted hand movements promptly disappeared as his attention was occupied. (I frequently have seen this type of primitive behavior in severely and profoundly retarded children who come from rather perplexed families, and who have received "the works" in diagnostic and/or treatment procedures.)

In my opinion, this type of emotionally disturbed/mentally retarded child essentially is an "untutored child" whose primitive behavior has been allowed to persist as the treatment focus of the
parents and professionals has been displaced into elucidation of fine
differential diagnostic issues and unrealistic curative-treatment interventions. The family slowly loses its tolerance and empathy for the
child as their initial high treatment/cure expectations and ongoing
investments of energy result only in slow dissolution of their hopes.

During a previous observation period, the child care workers at
this institution had begun to work actively with this youngster on
self-help skills and small group interactions and they showed rather
remarkable success! My treatment recommendations focussed upon
placing the diagnostic "merry-go-round" at rest, while stressing the
need for closer interpersonal relationships (e.g., foster-grandparent
contacts on a regular basis), continuity of similar passive-dependent
relationships and further involvement in a highly structured, developmentally oriented program to perfect self-help skills. Simultaneously, ongoing family interviews helped to clarify parental perplexity
and alter their demolished expectations of/from their child.

There is a lingering myth that retarded children—especially
the more severely retarded—must "look retarded." It would seem
that normal physical appearance in the presence of markedly
delayed muscular development and primitive behavior is viewed
as incongruous (and/or incompatible) both by lay and professional observers alike. However, the writer has examined a number of severely and profoundly retarded children who had won
photographic baby contests! Frequently, the appearance of such
children and the complexity of their family interpersonal transactions, against the backdrop of severe mental retardation, eventuates in the erroneous diagnostic impression of a psychotic disorder of childhood; a diagnosis wherein vastly different treatment-
management approaches are called for and different treatment
expectations or end-points are produced. Realignment of paren-
tal/professional expectations, clarification of diagnoses, and focus
upon specific treatment are the keys to providing effective help to
retarded individuals who display primitive behaviors.

ATYPICAL BEHAVIOR

Another frequently referred behavioral challenge is that of the
adolescent/young adult retardate who is committed to an institution because of ongoing adjustment difficulties within his home

community, but not necessarily within his primary family structure. Cardinal behaviors displayed by such retardates include poor control (as noted by emotional outbursts), impulsivity, sullenness, stubbornness, mild legal transgressions, and generally poor adaptations to prevocational or vocational training programs.

Psychiatric consultation most commonly is requested because: a) The youngster refuses to cooperate with the training or group social-living expectations of the institutional setting; or b) continual abrasive comments and/or contacts from the family belittle the institution's ability to help the individual family member. A result of such family conduct is the retardate's questioning, "Why was I put here?" and, "Why are you keeping me?" The family denies the reality of his social-adaptive problems while at the same time harassing the institutional staff for focussing upon and attempting positive modification of these problem behaviors.

These instances of "atypical behavior" are *only atypical for the institutional settings wherein this type of youngster finds himself* (i.e. they are really quite typical within the family and the specific primary subculture). Etiologic diagnosis usually is in the area of "cultural-familial mental retardation" or "idiopathic mental retardation." The psychiatric findings and family characteristics/adjustment tactics portrayed in the following case history are typical.

> The patient was a fourteen-year-old, mildly retarded boy whose parents had a common-law marriage. Delayed developmental milestones became more obvious when he entered school and increasing behavioral difficulties were noted. Later, a series of minor altercations with the police occurred, culminating in a car theft which necessitated his removal from the community. His parents tended to blame the school for his poor performance and subsequent maladjustment; institutionalization was very much against their wishes as they felt that they were being persecuted (e.g. "The law is against us." "He is a good boy if other folks will just leave him alone"). Adjustment to residential placement was characterized by frequent temper outbursts when demands were made upon him. He manifested continual sullenness and failed to involve himself in any of the institution's programs, except to demand that his parents be allowed to visit him weekly. Our basic concern was finding methods the staff might utilize to motivate him toward a more positive role in his ongoing training program.

In the case seminar, it became apparent that the staff minimized the importance of the family's anger toward the institution and the negative effect of their attitude upon their son's adjustment. Collectively, members of the treatment team provided information gleaned from letters, telephone calls, and family visits, all of which repeated the common theme that the family was not responsible for his placement, and continuing to convey the message, "You can come home whenever they will let you. . . ." It would have been extremely difficult for any individual staff member to be aware of the total clinical picture and associated treatment challenges. However, with clarification and direction, staff members were able to augment some imaginative intervention techniques. In a planned conference with both the parents and the boy present, the parents were told that they could take their son home if they so desired. The family responded by listing numerous factors which they would have to consider, then became quite uncomfortable and announced that they would telephone their decision to the boy. When the staff insisted that the boy be told of their decision in person and in the presence of staff members, the mother asked the boy to leave the room; she then stated that she couldn't tell him that she didn't want him to live at home because, "He will be mad at me." When the boy was told of the family's decision by the mother, he responded as predicted with an angry outburst directed toward his family. In the follow-up plan, the family's visits were restricted in number and to a member of the treatment team being present at all times. The boy's other contacts with his family, such as letters and telephone calls, were monitored. The staff was instructed to meet his angry outbursts with the disclaimer that they were there only to help him and were not holding him against the wishes of his family.

Cultural-familial mental retardation is almost ten times more frequent than all other causes of retardation combined, and yet 90 per cent of these cultural-familial retardates are not institutionalized. Those children who are institutionalized are placed for their own protection from severe emotional and material deprivation. Unfortunately, these children usually are the last to be identified as mentally retarded and already may have spent their formative years in deprived settings. Not only have they been identified with dyssocial and antisocial pathological living conditions, but their attitudes, defenses, and personality patterns usually are well entrenched by the time of institutionalization. Thus, the patient who is institutionalized within the general classification of cultural-familial mental retardation probably represents a specific subgroup of community problems.[2]

It would appear that institutionalized mentally retarded individuals with atypical behavior increasingly are "flunking out" of community based services programs and facilities to continue their persistently atypical behavior within a social system other than their primary family. Management is difficult unless very close coordination exists between the administrative segments of institutional treatment teams. In addition, professional staff countertransference problems are frequent and difficult in ongoing transactions with these patients and their families. For example, I frequently have noted highly restrictive punitive management approaches to these individuals, unnecessary utilization of psychoactive drugs (usually at high dosage levels), and terribly complex and confusing patterns of communication between the patient and his family, the patient and staff members, the family and staff members, the family and local politicians, etc. Yet it is in these very cases that the total treatment environment of an institutional setting can modify motivational potential, effect changes in the patient's value systems, and achieve more positive social-adaptive approaches to work and to interpersonal transactions. If these management dimensions are not explored and implemented, many retarded individuals with atypical behavior will again "flunk out," and possibly will become fixed dropouts from life itself.

Rather than focus only on the pathological spectrum of the "atypical behavior" group of individuals, the following case history illustrates the need to monitor closely the child's transition from his typical level of personality functioning within a closely knit family, to the atypical behavior he may manifest when placed in a residential treatment situation (e.g. an institution for the retarded, which is antithetical to his life style and his need for an emotional support system).

> The patient was a ten-year-old boy diagnosed as moderately mentally retarded resulting from a birth injury. He was the youngest of eight children of a closely knit middle-class family. Shortly after admission to an institution for the mentally retarded, the child refused to eat, became withdrawn and lost weight to a degree where there was medical concern for his survival. In brief, the clinical picture

was one of reactive "failure to thrive" with current indices to suggest further movement towards marked self-isolation and/or death. The parents had not visited since the time of admission, as they had been advised not to until he became "adjusted to institutionalization" (a routine admissions policy).

In the case seminar, the team recognized the need for extensive contact between the family and their boy, including ongoing counseling focussing upon the family's grief, and allowing a gradual separation. The family was also helped to realize that their boy did not have the capacity to handle or to totally understand the crisis of separation.

Children from closely knit families present a different therapeutic challenge than children from families where the intrafamilial relationship is secondary to extrafamilial concerns and activities (i.e. in sharp contrast to the first case history of the boy who displayed primitive behavior and whose family focussed upon their search for specificity of diagnosis, treatment methodology, and optimal prognosis rather than emotional interaction with their child!). Such children usually are admitted to an institution in late childhood, generally after prolonged empathic parental attempts to help them function effectively within the primary home setting. Often the family response to the child's need is marked to the degree that the total pattern of family functioning is organized around the care of the retarded child. In such instances, the child's personal and clinical history contains specific behavior patterns as well as the family's responses thereto, and this information provides the alert staff with guidelines for reducing the child's anxiety in a totally different situation, while simultaneously programming a series of gradual separation experiences for him. Such cases also serve as an excellent entrée into a review of the admissions procedures of the institution.

ABNORMAL BEHAVIOR

Abnormal behavior problems encountered by the author primarily have encompassed instances of psychotic behavior. It is truly remarkable that in the seventh decade of the 20th century, one still sees psychotic children who literally are dumped into institutions for the mentally retarded because of the lack of specific treatment programs in their home communities or because of the treatment nihilism of psychosis in early life. (This is a major problem as treatment is initiated, slowness of response wears out the treatment team, the child is referred as "untreatable," which is extrapolated to mental retardation with the prognosis "hopeless.") In the clinical interview, children with psychotic disorders present the following behavioral dimensions: a) bizarreness of manner, gesture and posture; b) uncommunicative speech; c) little or no discrimination between animate and inanimate objects (felt to be one of the primary signs of psychosis in childhood—an entity which is sharply delineated from the primitive behavior previously noted); d) identifies mostly with inanimate objects; e) displays deviant affective expressions; f) little, if any, relationship with peers; g) passive compliance to external demands or stimuli; and h) marked negativism (if pushed into an interpersonal setting, exhibits negativism, withdrawal, and out of contact behavior, i.e. psychosis).

Since the psychotic reactions of childhood noted in mentally retarded children have been discussed extensively elsewhere,[4, 6] they will not be commented upon further at this time. Rather, two case histories will be presented: The first to illustrate features of a psychotic reaction in late adolescence; and the second to show an instance of abnormal behavior which, though technically not classified as a psychosis, is truly an instance of abnormal behavior because the child is so out of touch with the world around him—the rumination syndrome.

> The patient was a nineteen-year-old farm boy who had been institutionalized at age seven because of frequent temper tantrums, noisy screeching, carrying a large screwdriver at all times and cruelty to animals. Personal history stated that at age three he was considered somewhat precocious by his parents, but was noted to display periodic elective mutism and a hearing loss was suspected. Shortly thereafter he became mute and regressed in his intellectual and motor achievements. At the time of admission he was considered "different and slow" and was quite unable to function in available special education options. The team was concerned about his withdrawal as well as his bizarre behavior, reporting that he watched the linoleum tile patterns quite carefully, turning to the right on every twenty-second tile interval. On direct examination he grimaced frequently, bizarre hand movements were evident, and he mumbled incoherently to himself. The diagnosis was mental retardation secondary to a major psychiatric disorder, childhood psychosis.[8]

A treatment plan, which included the use of psychotropic drugs and provision of a milieu which focussed on activities and closer interpersonal contacts, was devised for this patient. The chronicity of the boy's psychosis and his interpersonal unavailability was approached via the behavior modification paradigm[5] with focus on reestablishing both self-help skills and interpersonal contacts. Specific management foci included developing a repertoire of skills which would permit him to function in a less restrictive environment (e.g. a community based sheltered workshop and/or a residential hostel facility).

In cases of childhood psychosis, such an endpoint is far more normal and provides much greater personal fulfillment than the passive participation in an endless merry-go-round of residence in an institution for the mentally retarded followed by referral to a mental hospital and then assignment to yet another institution for the mentally retarded. Many institutions for the retarded have built up large backlogs of psychotic patients whose definite treatment needs have gone unmet to date! These patients are referred elsewhere during their acute episodes, then are returned in a subacute remission state. Since institutional staff personnel view these psychotic patients as "odd or dangerous," often the individual patient's psychotic process is refueled by staff members until he is precipitated once again into an acute state.

Despite the availability of accurate diagnostic techniques, it is not unusual for this type of patient to be institutionalized on an expediency basis. Therefore, the wide spectrum of treatment modalities for such patients mandate the formulation and provision of both general and specific therapies once diagnosis has been confirmed.

ABNORMAL (LIFE-THREATENING) BEHAVIOR

The occurrence of rare syndromes is interesting to observe, rather easy to describe, but difficult to interpret. The *rumination syndrome* in mentally retarded children illustrates these principles. The writer's experiences suggest that rumination may not be due to the mechanism of a psychosomatic disorder secondary to sustained emotional deprivation in early childhood, and/or failure of the individual mothering-in relationship.[11] In fact, the author has noted specific extrinsic factors which precipitate this syndrome in mentally retarded children. Rumination can be defined as bringing previously ingested food up into the mouth; a process which generally requires considerable effort on the part of the child, either by manipulation of the tongue and muscles of the throat or by putting the fingers into the mouth. The ability to ruminate evolves over a period of time, and, in its early manifestations is often mistaken for vomiting and is viewed as a possible symptom of gastrointestinal pathology. In many cases, rumination is associated with behavioral disturbances such as autistic posturing, excessive genital and fecal play, body-rocking, head-banging, and excessive thumb/finger sucking.

> The patient was an eight-and-one-half-year-old boy living in an institution for the mentally retarded. His personal history revealed that he was born after a normal pregnancy to a 31-year-old mother. At birth, he was noted to have multiple congenital anomalies, as manifested by absence of the left eye, skull asymmetry, webbing of the toes and hypospadia. Early in childhood, his slow developmental course and partial vision coupled with a psychologist's impression of moderate mental retardation, led the family physician to recommend institutionalization. As they lived in a rural community with little prospect for special education for their son, the family reluctantly agreed to institutionalization when the boy was three years old. This child experienced no appetite or weight problems while living in his own home. Within a week after entering the institution, he was described as quite restless, which was followed by a period of frequent crying and screaming. This behavior persisted for the first two months of institutionalization. His parents considered taking him back home, but were reassured that, "He'll get over it; he'll learn to like us; he seems so retarded that I don't think he really understands whether he's at home or not." During the initial periods of emotional upset, the child's appetite pattern became rather irregular, but he did not lose weight. During the remainder of the first year of institutionalization, he commonly was described in nursing notes as "quiet, sad looking, likes to play around with his tongue and his food, but seems to eat enough to get along." However, during the following year distinct rumination features were described; he became a feeding problem and slowly began to lose weight. Interestingly, the ward personnel recognized and were empathic with the child's increasing adverse reactions to institutional life and appointed one of the older girl residents to be his exclusive "feeder and leader." His rumination ceased within a month, and he became more outgoing and demanding, enjoyed playing in the ward sand-

box and on the outdoor recreational equipment. When we were asked to see him, the staff was quite concerned about the return of his former pattern of sadness, playing with his food and rapidly declining weight. On examination, rumination was very much in evidence, the child's gaze was averted and his behavior was autistic with much psychomotor slowing. A review of the total clinical situation revealed that the child's daily "feeder and leader" had been placed in a vocational rehabilitation program three months previously, and the replacement had attempted to fulfill her duties to the child rather mechanically. We discussed the boy's problems with his new helper, and it became apparent that his cosmetic handicaps, low developmental level and dependency/demandingness all had became rather repugnant to her. She complained bitterly about his "playing games with me with his food; if I get it down, he brings it back up; then he seems to have fun just chewing it and staring at me with a funny look on his face; like he's laughing at me or something."

In this particular instance, the child's former rumination phenomenon appeared to reactivate with changes in his interpersonal environment and the markedly altered relationship with his primary care giver. We were considering replacement of the child's second helper by another young lady (with attributes similar to his first helper), when his mother became very interested in his recent feeding problems. In view of newly established community outpatient facilities for the moderately retarded in their home town, she asked to take her son home with her. We discussed with her the essence of the foregoing clinical information, reviewed the boy's therapeutic needs and supported her interest in and relationship with her child. On last report (six months after discharge), the child was living at home, doing very nicely and had no further appetite or feeding problems (i.e. rumination).

The behavioral manifestations of young mentally retarded children most frequently have been described as developmentally delayed and in keeping with their general levels of endowment. Apparently, sufficient attention has not been directed toward the primitive, atypical, and abnormal behavioral manifestations of severely and moderately retarded young children, even though such behavior is encountered frequently.[7, 9, 10] In the past, manifestations of symptomatic behavior in mentally retarded children (such as head-banging and autistic hand play) were viewed as part of the underlying retardation process itself.[1] However, as has been demonstrated, behavioral manifestations (such as chronic head-banging in severely retarded children) are related to external environmental factors and can be modified or removed.[3]

It is interesting to note that the child with a rumination syndrome appears to be somewhere in between all three of the types of behavioral disturbance described in this chapter. Therefore, the author suggests that the psychiatrist utilize a variety of treatment techniques, many of which were specifically discussed in the previous sections on management of primitive, atypical, and abnormal behaviors. The more global treatment-management guidelines will be discussed in the following section.

TREATMENT-MANAGEMENT GUIDELINES

The number of emotionally disturbed mentally retarded individuals who are being admitted to institutions for the mentally retarded is increasing rapidly. Since these emotionally disturbed retardates so often are rejects from community based programs, they present a major challenge to members of the professional staff. A major evolving role of institutions for the mentally retarded is to provide regional resource programs and facilities to back up community based programs. Such redirection demands that the focus of professional staff members be tuned in sharply to behavioral dimensions of mental retardation and the needs of families who literally have been worn out by the primitive-atypical-abnormal behavior of their mentally retarded sons and daughters.

In the case of many individuals who present mental retardation and emotional disturbance, undue focus on one or the other of these personal developmental handicaps beclouds the issue of individual treatment needs and the sequence for providing same. Undue focus on singular diagnostic approaches will literally send such children on a merry-go-round of mental retardation facilities, mental health facilities, additional clinicians to confirm and reinforce diagnoses, etc.

Administrators are faced with decisions such as: a) Not providing psychiatric services, b) providing psychiatric consultation, c) implementing a psychiatric ward setting, or d) energetically attempting to weed out retardates with emotional problems and sending them to the mental health people. Although each of these particular administrative postures have been utilized in the different settings where the author has been employed, it would appear that none of them make very much sense in view of the rising number of emotionally disturbed retardates, the institutional and community based resources currently available and changing professional attitudes toward providing help for these individuals. I suggest the following guidelines for the professional who provides human management services for the emotionally disturbed mentally retarded individuals residing in an institutional setting.

Psychiatric diagnosis of the mentally retarded tends to become enmeshed in rather fruitless arguments concerning the etiologies of the individual's emotional disorder. The conceptual jump between diagnosis and prognosis is accomplished too rapidly, without any consideration of what treatment should be initiated, or whether or not any treatment should be administered. As noted in the case histories, equating diagnosis with prognosis may lead the professional literally to not suggest any treatment methodology! In contrast, I would suggest that the emotionally disturbed mentally retarded individual be evaluated based upon the known, principal, possibly causative factors in the evolution of his current disorder, a thorough description of his current behavior—stressing the type of disorder (i.e. primitive, atypical, or abnormal) and then outlining specific treatment-management goals. Specific goals not only are based on current diagnostic findings, but also on the long-range considerations such as: What is the future placement for this child? Can he return to his home, or is the door literally closed to him? Is treatment aimed at his current level of disorder designed so that he will be less disturbed, or that he will be less disturbing to institutional personnel? Long-range treatment goals are as important as short-range ones, because when the patient improves to the degree that there is no advancement program for him either in the institution or in the community, what motivation is there for him to maintain his improved behavior? Similarly, behavioral improvement without opportunity for developmental advancement (either in the institutional setting or in the community) will tend to have a negative effect on the morale of treating personnel who come to realize that their efforts to help the patient only result in his transfer from Building A to Building C. In other words, they see little hope that their positive efforts at behavior-shaping will extend into a series of developmental transactions in the outside world (e.g. in developmental day care, graduation to a workshop setting, or sheltered hostel living arrangement). The expectations and morale of treatment personnel must be stressed, for when the fruit of their labors becomes lost no long-lasting treatment-management results will be noted in their patients.

The previously reviewed descriptive diagnostic considerations and specific treatment-management plans strongly suggest that a variety of treatment approaches must be utilized to help the emotionally disturbed-mentally retarded individual. A mentally retarded individual with a psychotic disorder may need a specific ward or milieu setting, ongoing foster grandparent contacts, behavior-shaping to stimulate positive reinforcement of specific adaptive behaviors, psychoactive drugs to initiate reduction of motor and/or mood overactivity, involvement of the family support system, etc. Due to the complexity of these treatment ingredients, the team approach is the only meaningful way to provide a wide spectrum of individualized services for the emotionally disturbed/mentally retarded population.

SUMMARY

The increasing admission rate of emotionally disturbed/mentally retarded individuals to institutions for the mentally retarded demands a reevaluation of the individuals so referred, how they are evaluated, and the spectrum of treatment-management modalities that are available for them therein. The three most common emotional disturbances noted in institutionalized mentally retarded individuals have been presented. Specific treatment-management approaches for each of these types of emotional disturbance have also been presented.

Last, the administrative implications and suggested guidelines for implementing diagnostic and treatment approaches to these emotionally disturbed retarded individuals are presented within the context of redirected goals for institutions for the mentally retarded: as regional resource services for community-based programs for the mentally retarded.

REFERENCES

1. Barr, M. W.: *Mental Defectives: Their History, Treatment and Training.* Philadelphia, Pa., Blakiston's Son and Co., 1904.
2. Benda, C. F., Squire, N. D., Ogonik, J., and Wise, R.: Personality factors in mild mental retardation. Part I. Family background and socio-cultural patterns. *Am J Ment Defic,* 68:28-40, 1963.
3. Collins, D. T.: Head-banging: Its meaning and management in the severely retarded adult. *Bull Menninger Clin,* 29(4):205-211, 1965.
4. Eaton, L. and Menolascino, F. J.: Psychotic reactions of childhood: A follow-up study. *Am J Orthopsychiat,* 37:521-529, 1967.
5. Gardner, W. I.: Use of behavior therapy with the mentally retarded. In Menolascino, F. J. (Ed.): *Psychiatric Approaches to Mental Retardation.* New York, Basic Books, Inc., 1970. pp. 250-275.
6. Menolascino, F. J.: Psychoses of childhood: Experiences of a mental retardation pilot project. *Am J Ment Defic,* 70:83-92, 1965.
7. Menolascino, F. J.: Emotional disturbance and mental retardation. *Am J Ment Defic,* 70:248-256, 1965.
8. Menolascino, F. J.: Psychiatric findings in a sample of institutionalized mongoloids. *J Ment Subnorm,* 13:67-74, 1967.
9. Mowrer, O. H.: *Learning Theory and Behavior.* New York, John Wiley & Sons, 1960.
10. Webster, T. E.: Problems of emotional development in young retarded children. *Am J Psychiat,* 120:34-41, 1963.
11. Wright, M. M., and Menolascino, F. J.: Nurturant nursing of mentally retarded ruminators. *Am J Ment Defic,* 71:451-459, 1966.

Chapter 7

BEHAVIOR PROBLEMS OF THE MENTALLY RETARDED

Nathan B. Miron

A N individual is considered to be "mentally retarded" if his IQ falls below a given cutting score on various standardized tests. On one such test,[35] the IQ of 69 defines the upper limit of "retardation"; according to this test, IQ below 70 includes 3 per cent of the population of the United States. Using data of the 1970 census, and the criterion of the Stanford Binet, there would thus be about 6,000,000 mentally retarded individuals in the United States. This corresponds roughly to the combined populations of Chicago, Los Angeles, and Washington, D.C. By the same criterion, there would be 591,500 mentally retarded persons in California alone. On the other hand, there are only 14,370 mentally retarded people in state and private institutions in California,[40] including foster homes, family care, etc. Thus, in California alone, there are over 577,000 retarded people *not* in institutions; for every mentally retarded individual who is institutionalized in California, there are more than 40 who are not. It is assumed that these figures are roughly representative of the entire country.

Obviously, selection factors other than IQ are being employed in the process of institutionalization. Even though measurement along this dimension breaks down in the lower categories, the severity of retardation (roughly corresponding to IQ scores) does, in fact, play some role in selection. Society at large tends to find the severely retarded child or adult less appealing than one who is only mildly retarded, and the profoundly retarded are

The Sonoma State Hospital (Eldridge, California) studies of self-injurious behavior were under partial support of NIMH Research Grant No. 2R01 MH 15000-03, from the Center for Studies of Suicide Prevention of the National Institute of Mental Health.

often so grossly damaged that they require twenty-four-hour nursing care merely to stay alive. A large portion of the institutionalized retarded are not, however, in this category. Rather, they have been placed in institutions because of various behavior problems. The fact that they are also mentally retarded is only partly coincidental, inasmuch as the label "mentally retarded" implies a limited behavioral repertoire. This limited repertoire is why their test scores were so low in the first place. Given such extremely narrow behavioral repertoire, it follows that the retarded person has fewer means at his disposal for fulfilling his needs. In other words, his skills in obtaining reinforcers are very limited.

The basic needs of survival, such as food, clothing, and warmth are, of course, furnished—usually not contingent on the behavior of the individual. Thus, unlike most individuals outside of institutional walls, the retarded person traditionally does not have to pay for his meals, bed, clothing, or any of the basic implements of survival, either with money or with labor. On the other hand, his other needs, especially social, are very often not to be gratified under any circumstances. It should surprise no one that for years institutionalized individuals have often led lives which are drab, boring, and monotonous. It is well known that stimulus (sensory) deprivation and lack of pattern differentiation can result in rather extensive and disorganized behavioral changes.[6, 32] Social interactions in institutions for the retarded are often infrequent and superficial; interactions between staff and the retarded person often take place in a mechanical and routine, assembly-line fashion. Yet, if even these interactions are all a retarded person can look forward to, year after year, the attention of the staff becomes a sought-after commodity. This seems to be true even when the staff interact only to deliver aversive stimuli, such as commands, angry shouts, or even physical violence. It is a basic law of economics that when a commodity is in short supply and almost unlimited demand, individuals in the society will compete for that commodity. In the typical state institution, staff attention is in short supply and great demand. Many patients do indeed compete for attention. The situation is aggravated by chronic staffing shortages, and by reductions in the already short supply. Moreover, the limited staff must carry out numerous other duties which they consider important, such as functional nursing, including janitorial duties, setting up the dining room for meals, cleaning the dining room afterward, preparing medications, writing notes in the chart, repairing clothing of the patients, carrying out and picking up laundry, and answering telephones which ring endlessly. As a result, even a ward which is relatively richly staffed may assign a very low priority to programs which work with the patient to increase his level of development. The developmental progress of the institutionalized patient therefore tends to be still slower than one should expect or have reason to tolerate.

As a final difficulty, the few staff members who are available must be divided among three shifts, on a seven-day a week rotating basis. The end-result is usually from forty-five to one hundred patients on a ward, supervised by a small handful of staff. As many parents can testify, taking care of one or two children can be a full-time job, and professional people such as schoolteachers often throw up their hands when they are given classes even as large as 35 or 40 students.

The retarded person frequently learns how to obtain the attention of the staff in some way, usually by emitting behavior which is aversive to them. In general, staff members, in much the same manner as parents, teachers, law-enforcement agents, clergymen, and military leaders, tend to take "good" behavior for granted, and thus tend not to respond to it. On the other hand, they rather quickly react to behavior which they do not like. Thus, retarded persons learn that while they are "good," the staff tends to ignore them, taking advantage of the peaceful orderliness to do other chores, or simply to relax and take it easy. But "bad" behavior is frequently rewarded by attention and/or acquiescence to demands. Even a severely retarded child may learn in a remarkably short time that behavior problems (i.e. behaviors someone dislikes) usurp the priorities of staff time and effort. I have seen innumerable instances of ward life which was calm and tranquil, until a patient attacked another patient, beat himself, or created a similar emergency, sometimes with the aid of feces. In many cases, the staff responded immediately. They abandoned whatever they were doing, and moved quickly to intervene, to separate the patients, to scrub the walls, or to forcibly restrain the self-injurious patient. Time and again, patients who were quietly playing alone, or quietly walking around, disturbing nobody, were allowed to continue these activities for hours upon end, with seldom a glance from the staff. But within seconds of the onset of disruptive behavior, as many as five or six staff members focussed their attention upon the child with the offending behavior—sometimes for periods up to an hour for each incident.

The staff member then lives his entire professional life going from crisis to crisis. The child, in turn, lives his life creating crises for the staff. The behaviorist could well paraphrase Shakespeare by saying, "The evil that men do is reinforced; the good is oft' extinguished with their bones." No matter how one may wish to deny it, behavior problems *are* often followed by attention or other reinforcers, while acceptable behaviors *are* often ignored. Staff members thus find themselves in a vicious circle, in which they spend a major part of their time and effort unwittingly teaching and strengthening the behaviors of which they themselves approve the least. Fielding[11] commented, "The more you focus on an undesirable behavior and attend to it, the higher is the probability that the behavior will be emitted again. Especially, in a place where the average child is probably touched about four or five times a day."

Because behavior problems are so often instrumental in bringing the retarded individual to the hospital, and for keeping him there; and because they are a major source of distress to the staff; hospital workers spend an inordinately large amount of time in attempts to deal with them.[23] Thormahlen[36] reported that 37 per cent of staff time promoted dependence—a problem because it guarantees too low a limit on already limited skills. Much time is also spent indirectly in consultations, ward team meetings, and other procedures, often devoted specifically to their worst behavior problems. These meetings often tie up most of the ward staff simultaneously, thus aggravating the need for more staff members. The priority attached to behavior problems is illustrated by the author, who has spent a major part of the past three years in a Federally-funded project whose primary function has been to deal with a single behavior problem—self-injurious behavior (SIB).

Undesirable behavior among the mentally retarded is basically no different from undesirable behavior in the community at large. Often, in both cases, acceptable behavior is either ignored, reinforced insufficiently, or punished outright. In both cases, the problem behavior is receiving reinforcement on a schedule sufficiently frequent to maintain it. Often, in both cases, those in control of the community or ward rely upon punishment or threat of punishment in order to suppress undesirable behavior, with little thought given to the more important problem of shaping and maintaining desirable behaviors which could replace the behavior problem.

An important difference, however, lies in the circular fact, mentioned previously, that the retarded start out with major behavioral deficits; because they are retarded, there are few behavioral alternatives available to them. A person with a wide behavioral repertoire can try many ways of achieving thwarted goals. If we do not get what we want, we may use words to ask for it; we may buy it with tokens—the money we have earned because of our special abilities. We may plead; we may connive, lie, reason, write our congressman, or indulge in an extremely rich variety of behaviors, limited largely by our ingenuity. The retarded have few such options. Consequently, when a retarded person is rewarded by one of the few behaviors in his repertoire, he will be more likely to attempt the same strategy the next time conditions are similar. Where few choices are available, the successful behavior becomes reinforced all the more strongly, and the behavior is much more likely to perseverate. Further, many or perhaps all retarded have central nervous system damage which may increase the likelihood of perseveration. Add to this a situation in which the reinforcement is intermittent, and the result may be an extremely persistent problem, which could possibly be sustained for the remainder of the retarded person's life.

Behavior problems appear to be of three major types. The most obvious are behaviors of which a single occurrence is dangerous (e.g. biting), offensive (e.g. fecal smearing), or behaviors which are not considered problems until their rate becomes sufficiently high that someone becomes annoyed (e.g. stereotyped chattering). The common element among all behaviors of this type is that the behavior occurs too often. Because this type of problem is the most obvious, it has received the most attention, both on the ward and in the literature of behavior modification. The strategy employed or attempted is one of reducing the rate (i.e. frequency) or intensity of a behavior (e.g. SIB) to a level which does not appear to be harmful to the patient or others, and can be tolerated by the staff. Often, reduction of the intensity automatically accompanies the lower rate.[7, 26] This category includes tantrums, aggression toward others, prolonged screaming, toilet accidents, food throwing, stealing, deliberate property damage, and innumerable other behaviors, many of which are essentially attention-getting devices. In technical terms, contingent attention reinforces the behavior and maintains its rate.

A second type of behavior problem involves an insufficiently high rate of desirable behaviors. Thus, a retarded child may know how to eat with utensils, but may choose instead to eat with his hands, for reasons of his own (perhaps efficiency). He may be "nonambulatory," even though he knows how to walk, because instead of walking he chooses locomotion by scooting, or by holding up his arms—a response which has often been reinforced when a staff member or visitor picks up the child and carries him to his destination. While the problems of the first and second type are similar, they are described separately because the treatment strategies may be different. Thus, while most staff members will consider sloppy, hand feeding a problem (of the first type) they might not recognize that the problem may be reduced not only by the more obvious, common device of punishing hand feeding, but also by increasing the rate of utensil feeding; that scooting may be decreased not only by punishing scooting but by reinforcing walking. In brief, although the rate of a behavior may be decreased by punishing the behavior and by withdrawing the maintaining reinforcer, it may also be reduced by reinforcing alternative behaviors incompatible with the offending behavior.

Finally, a third category of behavior problem is the behavioral deficit. This is the least obvious, although possibly the most important from the long-range point of view, since a limited behavioral repertoire may set the stage for problem behaviors of the first two types. Behavioral deficits may make these problem behaviors necessary or valuable to the retarded person because they limit the number of ways in which an individual may obtain reinforcers. Where a problem behavior has functioned to funnel reinforcers this way, the probability is decreased that the retarded individual will find socially acceptable substitutes. In all likelihood, socially acceptable behaviors will not serve the purpose quite so well, since they may not so readily result in reinforcement.

Because the behavioral deficit is not a visible behavior, it often escapes notice of the staff. Sometimes, the deficit is recognized, but minimized or ignored, because the staff, not recognizing the significance of the role the deficit plays in generating behavior problems of the first type, assigns priority to reducing undesirable behaviors which are already present. Obnoxious behaviors have a way of intruding upon the attention of the staff, so that their presence is not likely to escape notice. This is in fact the patient's deliberate intention, in many cases. It is somewhat easier to recognize the presence of undesirable behaviors and then have meetings and consultations, or take other actions in hopes of reducing them, than it is to seek out and shape valuable new behaviors which are not yet in the repertoire of the patient.

Effectively increasing the behavioral repertoire requires some knowledge of developmental psychology, behavior analysis, and behavior modification, which many staff members do not have in their own repertoires. Although behavioral deficits are not always obvious, they are the essence of retardation. Nevertheless, partly because of the preoccupation with existing behavior problems of the first type, and partly because the staff is not yet aware of recent developments in the field of behavior modification, a circularity develops, which effectively limits the further development of the institutionalized patient: a patient with many behavioral deficits is first described as retarded because of his behavioral deficits. Once the label of retardation has been attached to the patient, staff members become convinced that the patient cannot be taught new behaviors—that because of his "retardation," he is incapable of further learning. Therefore, few attempts are made to enlarge his repertoire. Special education programs often bypass the patients with the most severe deficits, quite naturally choosing instead to work with higher-level patients—

those felt to be more "capable of learning." It is often stated that the "educable" retarded "have a greater potential," and thus the implication is that they are somehow more worthy of staff time and effort than are the severely retarded, who "cannot learn anyway." Moreover, the behavior problems associated with the latter are especially vexing to the staff, who may perhaps be pardoned for ignoring those who furnish them with so little success or other reinforcers.

Behavior problems of the first type may be reduced by either of three devices, or combinations of two or more of the three. The most common, punishment, refers technically to an event—usually, but not always aversive—which follows a given behavior and results in the reduction of its rate.*

A second device, extinction, refers to the systematic withdrawal of events which had in the past reinforced a given behavior, maintained its rate or increased it. A common example of extinction is simply ignoring a behavior when it happens.

Finally, the rate of a given behavior may be reduced by the reinforcement of responses which are incompatible with the behavior. This technique has already been mentioned in connection with hand feeding, scooting, etc.

Spectacular applications of behavior modification techniques in reducing behavior problems have been in the literature for a number of years. Although some of these examples have described projects with individuals not classified as retarded, many of the techniques are similar enough that highly successful results have been obtained when the procedures have been extrapolated to the retarded population. For example, "time-out," as applied by Wolf, *et al.*,[39] to problems of the first type with an autistic child, have worked well with the retarded, as will be described shortly.

PUNISHMENT

Application of aversive stimuli contingent to the occurrence of a given behavior is probably one of the most commonly attempted means of controlling behavior, and is loosely referred to as

---

* Punishment is not to be confused with negative reinforcement, which is a means of *increasing* the rate of a behavior by withdrawal of consequences (usually aversive) already present.

"punishment," whether or not it is successful (i.e. reduces the "punished" behavior). There is considerable question as to its effectiveness, both on theoretical and experimental grounds. As early as 1938, Skinner reported that the effects of aversive stimuli delivered to rats following bar pressing for food were temporary. These results have been supported by later studies, both in the animal laboratory[9] and in the clinic.[22] On the other hand, Solomon[33] disagreed, and cited a number of studies in which contingent application of aversive stimuli were indeed effective in reducing the rate of a behavior on a more or less permanent basis. Lovaas, *et al.*[16] reported that immediate contingent application of a harmless but distinctly painful electric shock quickly eliminated SIB, and that the behavior did not return after a follow-up period of eleven months. Azrin[1] reported animal studies which suggested that as the intensity of the aversive stimulus was increased, so was the probability that the behavior upon which it was contingent would be completely and permanently suppressed.

Threat of punishment is sometimes used to suppress behavior and results in setting up competing behaviors which tend to postpone or avoid the occurrence of the aversive stimulus. It should be pointed out, however, that where threats are effective, the reason may not be so much that the behaviors themselves were being punished directly, but rather that competing avoidance behaviors have been reinforced. It has been well established that postponement of aversive stimuli may reinforce behaviors which resulted in the avoidance.[30] Unfortunately, avoidance behavior tends to extinguish if the aversive stimulus is not occasionally presented.[29]

Clinical applications of aversive conditioning to the behavior problems of the retarded have received a great deal of attention in recent years. Among the earliest applications was that of Lovaas, *et al.*[16] using a contingent aversive stimulus (shock) to reduce SIB and bizarre behavior in autistic children, closely followed by Banks and Locke,[5] who temporarily reduced SIB by using an aversive consequence (hair pulling). Hamilton and Standahl[13] reduced screaming in a retarded adult girl. Luckey, *et al.*[18] and White and Taylor[38] used contingent electric shock to reduce vomiting and inappropriate food rumination with retarded patients.

For the past three or four years, the author has worked with self-injurious severely retarded children at Sonoma State Hospital, California's largest institution for the mentally retarded. During the course of this work, more than ten severely self-injurious patients have received strong electric shock contingent upon SIB. In every case, the rate of the behavior was drastically reduced.[22] In some cases the patients had regularly hit themselves, with considerable violence, as many as 20,000 times in a single day. One severely retarded fourteen-year-old girl produced approximately 4,000 SIB per day. Following use of contingent shock, the observed rate of SIB was reduced to approximately twenty-five light taps observed during a period of six months, although it is possible that several unobserved occurrences took place. However, in every child, SIB eventually returned, although not always to its former rate. Our experience suggests that the use of contingent aversive stimuli is considerably trickier than other devices, although because of the immediate, though temporary, reduction of SIB, its use is sometimes strongly indicated.

EXTINCTION

As mentioned before, extinction refers to the decrease in response rate contingent upon removal of events which had maintained the behavior. Removal of reinforcers has an essential simplicity which makes it appealing, both from a theoretical and practical point of view. If the reinforcers which maintained a behavior are not withdrawn, even though a behavior is followed by intensely aversive consequences, conflicting forces may be set up. It makes little sense to "punish" a behavior in order to reduce its rate when insufficient effort has been devoted to the elimination of the reinforcers which helped shape and maintain the behavior. Consequently, extinction is necessary, even when other means of rate reduction are employed.

The technique of Wolf, *et al.*,[39] isolation (time-out) contingent upon tantrum behavior, has been successfully employed by Lovaas, *et al.*[16] and Lovaas and Simmons[17] with autistic children, by Bostow and Bailey,[8] by Hamilton, Stephens, and Allen,[14] by Streifel,[34] and by Miron[20] with retarded patients. The technique is a simple one, in which SIB, tantrum, aggression, or other problem behaviors, were reduced by withdrawing the contingent atten-

tion which had previously reinforced them. The child was placed
in seclusion immediately upon the onset of the behavior, and no
social interactions with other people were allowed to take place
until the tantrum had run its course. Lovaas and Simmons[17]
found that these periods of non-attention (i.e. extinction) were
successful in eliminating SIB, although his periods of isolation
were scheduled for a specific length of time, and therefore were
not contingent upon the onset of SIB. On the other hand, attempts at Sonoma State Hospital to deal with SIB by placing the
child in isolation contingent upon the appearance of SIB were not
entirely successful.[22, 26] Although spectacular reductions in the
behavior occurred (see Fig. 3), subsequent "loosening" of the
rigor resulted in return of reinforcement for the SIB, and a
consequent rise in the rate. Moreover, SIB tended to come under
strong stimulus control.[26]

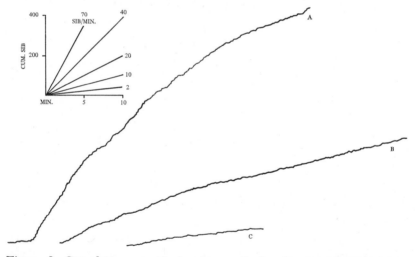

Figure 3. Cumulative record showing gradual reduction of SIB during
an extinction session. Each time a response occurs, a pen stepped upward,
tracing the curve upon a slowly moving paper strip. The scale is shown:
total number of SIB is shown on the ordinate, elapsed time on the abscissa,
and rate (SIB/minute) by the slope of the line. Five rates, from 2-70 SIB/
minute, are shown for comparison. The original record was divided into
three parts, to save space; curves B and C continue without pause from
curve A. In the record shown, approximately 1850 SIB occurred in 101
minutes; the initial rate of 70 SIB/minute decreased to a rate of 2 SIB/
minute by the end of C.

Retarded children were found to have very low rates (nearly zero) of SIB under some conditions (e.g. in certain rooms, or when a protective helmet was worn) and extremely high rates under other conditions. These rates may be as high as 16,000 to 20,000 hits per day in some locations. Lovaas and Simmons[17] later reported that stimulus specificity during extinction of SIB was also observed among their patients.

It is the view of the author that the effectiveness of time-out results from the fact that while the child is in seclusion, his tantrum may run its course with little danger of accidental social reinforcement. On the other hand, isolation does have its aversive properties for most individuals, and Wolf, *et al.*[39] regard "time-out" chiefly as a mild aversive stimulus. If the latter view is true, it suggests another interpretation for the rise in rate of SIB after the rate had been reduced by the "time-out." Many studies in punishment have demonstrated the return of a "punished" behavior when the behavior was no longer followed by aversive consequences.[1, 4]

It is wise to consider a few *caveats* before total commitment to an extinction program. First of all, immediately upon beginning extinction, a phenomenon sometimes called "behavioral contrast" may take place. Behavioral contrast refers to an increase in rate of a behavior or a surge of random behaviors just before the rate begins to decrease, following the withdrawal of customary reinforcers. Thus, when a parent or staff member decides that he will no longer pay his customary attention to the child who is engaged in tantrum behavior, he is often disappointed to observe that extinction does not take place at once. Rather, seemingly in an effort to obtain the usual, expected reinforcers for his tantrum, the child steps up his effort somewhat, and he may, for example, scream louder than usual. We have observed self-injurious retarded children, isolated in "time out rooms" where they could be observed through one-way mirrors or by video monitoring. Their rates gradually decreased, in the absence of social reinforcers, although there was often an initial spurt of behavior.

It is crucial that no reinforcement take place during the temporary period of higher rate, since this would serve to reinforce a higher rate of the behavior we wish to eliminate. It is possible that something similar to this takes place in the genesis of problems such as self-injury. Parents or staff may gradually "adapt" to a tantrum of a given level. The child, not receiving the reinforcers appropriate to that level of tantrum, begins another episode of tantrum, at a higher level (behavioral contrast). As the rate again increases, there is generally an increase in the intensity as well. Such increases often frighten the parent, who may eventually respond. The response, even when aversive, may reinforce the *higher* level SIB. In this way, by a series of successive escalations, in which the rate and intensity eventually exceed the threshold which can be tolerated, a minor problem may accelerate into a devastating one, a lesson not yet learned by leaders in the Pentagon.

A second *caveat* refers to the length of time necessary for extinction. It is well known that resistance to extinction is prolonged when the reinforcers which maintained a behavior are spaced rather infrequently, according to a variable schedule. A behavior which is reinforced every time it occurs is also most likely to disappear when the reinforcers are suddenly withdrawn. Why this is so is a mystery, but there is no question that this is the case.[10] A person drops a few coins into a soft-drink machine which, after long periods of reliable operation, suddenly fails to deliver the expected reinforcer. On the other hand, identical behavior, in front of a slot machine in Reno, may be extremely persistent. The slot machine delivers reinforcers on a random schedule, and a rather "thin" schedule (i.e. reinforcements widely spaced).

One need not set up elaborate shaping experiments in the laboratory in order to observe the effects of thin variable schedules of reinforcement. It is quite impressive when Skinner demonstrates a laboratory pigeon pecking a key over 73,000 times without a reinforcer.[10] The experimental laboratory is not the only place to observe the effects of variable schedules; such schedules maintain most behavior, both inside and out of institutions. Most behaviors in everyday life, especially in an institution, are probably reinforced rather randomly, and more or less infrequently. Those behaviors which survive become quite durable in the process, especially when viewed in the context of a meager repertoire of alternative behaviors. We have observed one retarded boy lightly bump his head against a door for a period of more than five and one-half hours. During this period, his head contacted the door more than 17,000 times, with no pause as long as thirty seconds.

This enormous resistance to extinction suggests that when the clinician decides to use extinction in order to eliminate a behavior, he had better be prepared to be very patient. Lovaas and Simmons[17] reported that extinction of SIB requires the patient make thousands of responses without social consequences. Our own results at Sonoma State Hospital have supported this finding.[20, 22]

Knowledge of the resistance to extinction and its functional relationship to the schedule under which the reinforcement was administered is valuable in yet another, more positive way. When new behaviors are being taught, resistance to extinction is often considered to be an asset, or a goal. One rarely tries to condition a new behavior if that behavior is not seen as desirable. It would be preferable if the desirable behaviors being taught became relatively permanent. Special effort should therefore be made to strengthen the new, desirable behaviors being deliberately shaped. Such strength comes from a thin variable schedule. While learning of new skills takes place most rapidly when reinforcement occurs on every appearance of the behavior, extinction at this time takes place in an incredibly short time. Usually, only two or three unreinforced repetitions of a new, weak behavior are required before extinction is more or less complete. Thus, desirable behaviors should initially be reinforced each time they occur, while they are still new and weak. Gradually, a single emission of the behavior should be allowed to go unreinforced; the next occurrence of the behavior is reinforced, before extinction has had the chance to occur. Some time later, another reinforcer is skipped, etc. If the number of consecutive unreinforced trials is not increased too rapidly, the schedule of reinforcement may be successfully thinned, by small increments. Should too rapid a tapering off take place during this crucial time, the result, of course, will be extinction, and the behavior simply disappears. The wise teacher will then recognize that he has made the most common error of the novice behavior modifier—that of impatience.

The novice may assume that the reinforcer is not effective because of insufficient deprivation. For example, he may assume food is not an effective reinforcer because the patient is not sufficiently "hungry" (i.e. food-deprived). The experienced behavior modifier will recognize instead that extinction has taken place, and that he must again start over, perhaps from the beginning, and repeat the entire shaping process. Fortunately, reshaping, as other relearning, generally takes less time than the initial shaping.

REINFORCEMENT OF INCOMPATIBLE BEHAVIORS

A third method of decreasing behavior is the reinforcement of incompatible behaviors: a child cannot sit and stand simultaneously. He cannot whisper and scream at the same time. He cannot be dressed and stripped at the same time. He cannot be in the northwest and southeast corners of a very large room at the same time. In short, there are many conditions which are mutually exclusive. By increasing the time spent sitting quietly, one may automatically decrease the time spent running around screaming, especially where the categories of mutually exclusive behavior comprise the universe of available responses. One may keep a person on one side of a line either by punishing him for crossing the line, or by reinforcing him for staying on his side of the line.

The third method is to be preferred, if implementation is at all practical, partly because of drawbacks in the other methods. Extinction takes a great deal of time and may be difficult to implement. Aversive control often generates counter-aggression;[2] "punished behavior" tends to return, once the aversive stimulus is withdrawn.[31] Moreover, it was mentioned earlier that the use of aversive conditioning results in somewhat unpredictable results. In any event, the world already seems too full of control by means of force. Both aversive control and extinction have the additional drawbacks that they do not systematically increase the behavioral repertoire of the patient. Such increases do occur when behaviors incompatible to the undesirable behaviors are reinforced. The staff member simply teaches a new behavior, and reinforces it when it occurs, with thinning of the schedule according to the explanation above.

Unfortunately, this method, desirable as it may be, is not always practical. First of all, as mentioned before, institutionalized children, as a function of the peculiar anthropology of the institution, tend to select behavior problems which leave the staff little choice. These behaviors are often genuine emergencies, and must be treated as such. Extinction of behavior problems and reinforcement of more desirable behavior incompatible with them take a great deal of time, which may not appear to be immediately available. Firemen in the middle of a raging forest fire give higher priority to extinguishing the blaze than lecturing to the public about Smokey the Bear! Despite this, however, the best time to work on emergencies is when they are *not* occurring.

Nevertheless, staff members often spend most of their time "putting out fires," rather than practicing "fire prevention." Again, SIB and aggression furnish examples which are quite common in institutions for the retarded. Few staff members would be prepared to isolate a child while he hit himself thousands of times, even though they were reinforcing alternative behaviors in the brief intervals of time between hits. The risks to the job of the staff member, to say nothing of the physical well-being of the child, are very real; and these risks would cause most staff members to rule out the treatment method, if indeed such a program had occurred to them at all. In addition, where the undesirable behavior is a repetitious one, occurring rapidly, the effects of the reinforcer may linger such a long time that a number of the undesirable behaviors may occur in the meantime, and be reinforced by it. Moreover, in some cases, no clear-cut alternative behavior occurs, other than the general category of "non-behavior." It is difficult, if not impossible, to reinforce a non-behavior. If we administer reinforcement to a person when he is not injuring himself, we are actually administering reinforcers at the time he is doing something else; the "something else" may be behaviors of an almost infinite variety. It is time-contingent, rather than behavior-contingent reinforcement, but some behavior must always be occurring at the time of reinforcement. Unfortunately, however, much of the time the behavior simply involves sitting quietly, "doing nothing." Thus, it is possible that vegetative behavior may be accidently shaped in the process.[24]

Finally, when a problem behavior occurs at an extremely low rate, reinforcement of incompatible behavior is not often successful in eliminating the residual behavior. For example, we observed a twenty-year-old severely retarded girl who would occasionally spring from her bench and hurtle across the room with her head lowered. She butted her head against the window panels, somehow judging precisely how hard to strike in order to break the window, yet bounce back with no injury to herself. Since other patients picked up the broken glass and ate it, the results were potentially hazardous to others, as well as to herself, and very expensive; she had broken more than a hundred panels. Her window-breaking occurred approximately twice weekly, at unpredictable times.

Conceivably, she could receive "high-density reinforcement"[3] and still continue to emit a behavior which occurred less than once a day. She would simply lose some reinforcers while breaking the window, but continue to obtain them when she did not. Whatever reinforcers maintained her window-breaking might still continue to do so.

As a practical matter, all three methods of eliminating behavior problems may be used in combination. Thus, it may be necessary at times to present aversive stimuli in order to reduce the rate and intensity of behaviors which constitute emergencies. One might ultimately teach a young child to stay out of the street by ignoring him when he is in the street and presenting social reinforcers, candy, or other goodies when he is not in the street. Aside from the fact that most parents rarely remember to reinforce out-of-the-street playing, the fact remains that if he is not quickly removed from the street, the entire training program could meet with a sudden and disastrous end. The use of a strong punisher might be the most practical treatment in such a case, as well as others which may come to mind. The most common mistake, however, is that when punishment is employed, the reinforcement of alternative behaviors is often forgotten, or rarely even considered. Each individual must have several options. If a behavior is punished, it should be mandatory that reinforcers be made available when acceptable alternatives, incompatible with the punished behavior, are emitted. Thus, a combination of punishment for the emergency, reinforcement of other, more desirable alternative behaviors, and a careful withdrawal of reinforcers for the punished behavior, may be employed. It makes little sense for a parent to spank a child and then spend the next ten minutes apologizing and kissing the child "for reassurance."

Peterson and Peterson[28] successfully reduced SIB by reinforcing periods of non-SIB with a blanket which appeared to be of great value to the child. If the child emitted no SIB during the criterion period, he was given his "Linus blanket," which he could not keep if SIB occurred. Wiesen and Watson[37] reinforced appropriate peer interaction in a retarded boy, while presenting aversive consequences for inappropriate attention-seeking behavior. Patterson[27] has developed a system of utilizing the peers of children with behavior problems to reinforce behavior incompatible with the problem behavior. An interesting and exciting feature of his system lies in its setting up subsystems which result in reinforcement for the peers when they reinforce behavior incompatible with the problem behavior. Although developed primarily in schools for "normal" children, the probability of its success with the retarded appears high.

Most of the common behavior problems of normal children also occur in the retarded child; the severity of the problems is somewhat compounded by the higher probability the child will be institutionalized, a process which seems to maximize the likelihood that behavior problems will occur and/or be maintained. The retardate, because of his meager repertoire of behaviors, is also less capable of developing alternatives.

No survey of the clinical applications of operant conditioning procedures would be complete without mention of the spectacular shaping procedures employed by Lovaas, *et al.* to teach speech to autistic children. With mute children, imitative speech was shaped, one sound at a time; sounds in the repertoire were then combined to form words, which were then imitated, upon request by the staff member. Ultimately, meanings were associated with the words, and functional sentences were built from the words. Gray and Fygetakis[12] also working primarily with non-retarded children, have specifically extended this type of speech training to include the functional use of correct grammar and syntax. An important feature of their program has been the construction of a number of individual programs, each based upon a symbolic logic model which utilized highly structured tasks, carefully graded in difficulty. Instructions for the staff were specifically designated, according to whether the child had performed the step correctly or incorrectly. Either of the binary choices—correct or incorrect—had predetermined consequences. This procedure enabled relatively untrained staff to implement the program as well as a trained psychologist or speech therapist could have done, merely by following all instructions literally.

Although neither of the last two studies dealt specifically with the mentally retarded, features of both have been applied to programs with severely retarded at Sonoma State Hospital, since the lack of speech is an important behavioral deficit. A fourteen-year-old severely retarded nonverbal girl was taught an imitative speech repertoire by a shaping procedure similar to that of Lovaas, *et al.*[15] (Miron[21]). The symbolic logic model of Gray and Fygetakis[12] has been applied to the reduction of SIB with severely retarded,[25] and toward the programming of speech training, reducing behavior problems, and increasing self-help skills.[19]

The preceding discussion should be considered a sampling of the literature describing applications of behavior modification principles to the behavior problems of the mentally retarded, and may be justly criticized for the sins of omission. The literature describing such applications has grown with extreme rapidity over the past five or ten years, and should continue to do so, as research and training continue to expand. It is through the recent systematic application of principles of behavior—notably operant conditioning—that the greatest strides in the treatment of the mentally retarded have been made. Generally speaking, through the systematic application of behavior modification principles, it has been possible to modify the behavior of patients with more severe handicaps and much more limited behavioral repertoires —the so-called "severely retarded," or "profoundly retarded." The shaping of complex skills in these individuals, the greater employment of subdoctoral staff in the "therapeutic process," and a "new look" on many wards have been some of the by-products of a system whose strongest features include making explicit the behavior to be modified, the treatment program itself, and the observed data resulting from the program. The self-monitoring which becomes possible by dependence upon observed data and the sensitivity which is thereby given to a treatment program contain the seeds of considerable promise of therapeutic developments still to come.

ACKNOWLEDGMENTS

Appreciation is especially expressed toward the administration of Sonoma State Hospital, including George Butler, M.D., Superintendent and Medical Director; Donald Dean, M.D., Program Director, Growth and Development Division; Charles McKean, M.D., Chief of Research; and Joseph O'Neill, former Superintendent and Medical Director (now at Siskiyou County Mental Health Services, California). In addition, we are deeply indebted and grateful to the competent, hard-working, and loyal nursing staff affiliated with ITU, both in the past and present, who carried out the bulk of the work associated with the studies. We thank the nursing administrative staff, especially Denver Henley, ASNS, ward charges Norine Kloeckner, PT II, George Daly, PT II, and acting ward charge Frank Venus, PT I. We also thank the enthusiastic and talented student professional assistants who took part in these studies, especially Royal Alsup, M.A., for helping read proof. Finally, the tireless efforts of Helen Hagerty, whose clerical and other contributions were far too numerous to catalog, have all been extremely vital.

REFERENCES

1. Azrin, N. H.: Effects of punishment intensity during variable-interval reinforcement. *J Exp Anal Behav*, 3:123-142, 1960.
2. Azrin, N. H.: Pain and aggression. *Psychol Today*, 1:26-33, 1967.
3. Azrin, N. H.: Presentation at Conference on Behavior Modification, Stockton, California, May 2, 1970.
4. Azrin, N. H.: Punishment and recovery during fixed-ratio performance. *J Exp Anal Behav*, 3:301-305, 1959.
5. Banks, M. and Locke, B. J.: Self-injurious Stereotypes and Mild Punishment with Retarded Subjects. *Parsons Research Project*, 1966. (Working Paper #123.)
6. Bexton, W. H., Heron, W., and Scott, T. H.: Effects of decreased variation in the sensory environment. *Canad J Psychol*, 8:70-76, 1954.
7. Boggs, L. J. and Miron, N. B.: Fixed Ratio Punishment in the Reduction

of Self-Injury in a Severely Retarded Boy. Paper read at the Convention of the California State Psychological Association, Los Angeles, 1972.

8. Bostow, D. E. and Bailey, J. B.: Modification of severe disruptive and aggressive behavior using brief time-out and reinforcement procedures. *J Appl Behav Anal*, 2:31-37, 1969.

9. Estes, W. K.: An experimental study of punishment. *Psychol Monogr*, 57, 1944 (3, Whole No. 263).

10. Ferster, C. and Skinner, B. F.: *Schedules of Reinforcement*. New York, Appleton-Century-Crofts, 1957.

11. Fielding, L. T.: A Presentation on the Guidelines for Operant Conditioning Applications. Address to Undergraduate Evening Psychology Colloquium Series. St. Cloud State College, St. Cloud, Minnesota, June 19, 1969.

12. Gray, B. B. and Fygetakis, L.: Mediated language acquisition for dysphasic children. *Behav Res Ther*, 6:263-280, 1968.

13. Hamilton, J. and Standahl, J.: Suppression of stereotyped screaming behavior in a profoundly retarded institutionalized female. *J Exp Child Psychol*, 7:114-121, 1969.

14. Hamilton, J., Stephens, L., and Allen, P.: Controlling aggressive and destructive behavior in severely retarded institutionalized residents. *Am J Ment Defic*, 71:852-856, 1967.

15. Lovaas, O. I., Berberich, J. P., Perloff, B. F., and Schaeffer, B.: Acquisition of imitative speech by schizophrenic children. *Science*, 151:705-707, 1966.

16. Lovaas, O. I., Freitag, G., Kinder, M. I., Rubenstein, D. B., Schaeffer, B., and Simmons, J. Q.: Experimental Studies in Childhood Schizophrenia: Developing Social Behavior Using Electric Shock. Paper read at the Convention of the American Psychological Association, Los Angeles, 1964.

17. Lovaas, O. I. and Simmons, J. Q.: Manipulation of self-destruction in three retarded children. *J Appl Behav Anal*, 2:143-157, 1969.

18. Luckey, R. E., Watson, C. M., and Musick, J. K.: Aversive conditioning as a means of inhibiting vomiting and rumination. *Am J Ment Defic*, 73:139-142, 1968.

19. Martin, P. L.: Technical Note: Community Behavioral Treatment Programs. In press, 1971.

20. Miron, N. B.: Modification of Self-Injurious Behavior in Severely Retarded Patients Through the Use of Operant Conditioning Techniques. Paper read at the Convention of the Western Psychological Association, San Diego, California, 1968.

21. Miron, N. B.: Shaping Imitative Speech in a Mute 14-Year-Old Severely Retarded Girl: A Brief Case Report. In press, 1971.

22. Miron, N. B. and Alsup, R. E.: Aversive Control of Self-Injurious Be-

havior of Institutionalized, Severely Retarded Children: Some Successes, Difficulties, and Failures. Paper read at the Convention of the Western Psychological Association, Portland Oregon, April, 1972.

23. Miron, N. B. and Daly, G.: A Cost-Accounting of Staff Time Spent in Response to Behavior Problems of Severely Retarded Children: Reduction of Cost by Behavior Modification Techniques. In press, 1971a.

24. Miron, N. B. and Daly, G.: Delayed Punishment in the Reduction of Self-Injurious Behavior in a Severely Retarded Girl. In press, 1971b.

25. Miron, N. B. and Daly, G.: Use of a Program Derived from a Symbolic Logic Model of Binary Choice, in the Reduction of Self-Injurious Behavior in Severely Retarded Children. In press, 1971c.

26. Miron, N. B. and Rooney, J. B.: The Accidental Acquisition of Stimulus Control During Extinction of Self-Injurious Behavior in a Severely Retarded Girl. Paper read at the Convention of the Western Psychological Association, Portland, Oregon, April, 1972.

27. Patterson, G. R.: Social Learning: An Additional Base for Developing Behavior Modification Technologies. In Frank, C.: *Assessment and Status of the Behavior Therapies and Associated Developments.* New York, McGraw-Hill Co., 1967.

28. Peterson, R. F. and Peterson, L. R.: The use of positive reinforcement in the control of self-destructive behavior in a retarded boy. *J Exp Child Psychol,* 6:351-360, 1965.

29. Sidman, M.: Avoidance Behavior. In Honig, W. K.: *Operant Behavior: Areas of Research and Application.* New York, Appleton-Century-Crofts, 1966.

30. Sidman, M.: Avoidance conditioning with brief shock and no exteroceptive warning signal. *Science,* 118:145-158, 1953.

31. Skinner, B. F.: *The Behavior of Organisms: An Experimental Analysis.* New York, Appleton-Century-Crofts, 1938.

32. Solomon, P., Kubzansky, P. E., Leiderman, P. H., Mendelson, J. H., Trumbull, R., and Wexler, D.: *Sensory Deprivation.* Cambridge, Harvard University Press, 1961

33. Solomon, R. L.: Punishment. *Am Psychol,* 4:239-253, 1964.

34. Streifel, S.: Isolation as a Behavioral Management Procedure with Retarded Children. Paper read at the 91st annual meeting of the American Association on Mental Deficiency, Denver, Colorado, 1967.

35. Terman, L. M. and Merrill, Maud A.: *Stanford-Binet Intelligence Scale, Form L-M.* Boston, Houghton Mifflin Co., 1960

36. Thormahlen, P. W.: A Study of On-the-Ward Training of Trainable Mentally Retarded Children in a State Institution. State of California, Department of Mental Hygiene, 1965. *(Research Monograph #4).*

37. Wiesen, A. E. and Watson, E.: Elimination of attention seeking behavior in a retarded child. *Am J Ment Defic*, 72:50-52, 1967.
38. White, J. C. and Taylor, D. J.: Noxious conditioning as a treatment for rumination. *Ment Retard*, 5:30-33, 1967.
39. Wolf, M. M., Risley, T., and Mees, H.: Application of operant conditioning procedures to the behavior problems of an autistic child. *Behav Res Ther*, 1:305-312, 1964.
40. Young, D. R. (Ed.): *Directory for Exceptional Children, 6th Ed.* Boston, Porter Sargent Co., 1969

Chapter 8

RESOCIALIZATION OF THE ACTING-OUT FEMALE RETARDATE

SHELDON R. GELMAN

THE treatment of the antisocial and aggressive retardate has increasingly received attention in recent publications. Specialized programs to treat and meet the demands of these behaviorally disturbed individuals have been established throughout the country (i.e. Murdock Center, North Carolina; Porterville State Hospital, California; Fairview Hospital and Training Center, Oregon; Johnstone Training Center, New Jersey; Rome State School, New York). An entire workshop at the 20th Mental Hospital Institute was devoted to this subject. It is clear that no agreement has been reached regarding the type of individual who falls into this broad descriptive category or the most effective treatment modality available. The only consensus that can be reached is that they present multiple problems. The following is a description of our experiences, problems, and observations working with a group of these individuals at the Laurelton State School and Hospital.

Laurelton State School and Hospital is one of nine institutions for the mentally retarded operated by the Commonwealth of Pennsylvania through its Department of Public Welfare.* Laurelton is unique among the state facilities for the retarded in that its rehabilitative program serves mildly and moderately retarded females of child bearing age from all sixty-seven counties of the Commonwealth. The majority of students admitted to Laurelton come from the large urban centers of Philadelphia and Pittsburgh. Students usually enter the institution in their mid-teens

* Under Pennsylvania's new Regionalization Plan Laurelton's focus was altered to that of a coed, regionalized, multi-purpose facility in July of 1969. The present report was prepared in December, 1968.

with the average length of stay being approximately three years. At any one time, there are approximately 700 students on the grounds and 325 students on community placement. Discharges average about 110 per year.

As an outgrowth of an in-service training program conducted during 1964-1965 (NIMH In-Service Training Grant, MH-10691-01), the staff of the Laurelton State School and Hospital developed a policy statement as to the goals and philosophy of the institution. In part, this statement viewed the major role of the institution as being rehabilitative with increased emphasis on returning individuals to the community as productive citizens. Such a statement coupled with a growing concern for the individual resident pointed out that a conflict existed between the presence of "untreated" individuals and the goals of rehabilitation and return to the community.

This "untreated" segment of the population was comprised of two major groups. To an increasing degree, new admissions to the institution were individuals whose major difficulty was not their retardation, but an inability to function appropriately in interpersonal situations (i.e. incorrigibility, truancy, promiscuity, disruptive and delinquent behavior). Their continued delinquent activities within the institution necessitated exclusion from available programs. The other "untreated" population was comprised of individuals who had been institutionalized for a number of years and had continually gotten into difficulty because of aggressive and acting-out behavior. They were labelled as "untreatable," and were permitted to remain as such.

THE READJUSTMENT UNIT

The problem of the "untreated" and "untreatable" individual reached a crisis level during September of 1965, with a sharp increase in acting out and destructive behavior. In October of 1965, the staff united in an attempt to reach these individuals with the establishment of an intensive treatment unit (readjustment unit).

The function of the readjustment unit was to attempt to alter unacceptable or irresponsible behavior on the part of our students through a controlled treatment-oriented environment. The readjustment unit was a locked, self-contained unit with an active treatment orientation. In more explicit terms, the goals and objectives of the cottage programs were as follows:

1. To help alter students' behavior from unacceptable to acceptable so that she might return to the community or to an open cottage.
2. To help students through difficult periods in their institutional adjustment.
3. To permit girls to work through their difficulties by expression and clarification of behavior within a controlled setting.
4. To teach methods for resisting frustration and achieving emotional control.
5. To outline standards of acceptable conduct within the abilities of each individual.
6. To help students learn to accept responsibility for their actions and behavior.
7. To help students make decisions by first thinking, then evaluating, and finally, taking action.
8. To stress the here and now of students' lives and what they are presently doing which is causing difficulty.
9. To build self-confidence and respect by providing experiences in which a student could be successful.
10. To help students accept the reality of their handicaps and to function to the best of their ability.
11. To provide a milieu which is stable, consistent, and could meet the needs of the students being referred.
12. To serve as a treatment tool rather than a means of punishment for the residents of the unit whose needs were such that they could not adjust in the regular institutional population.

We were reluctant to place a descriptive label on our population in that they appeared to possess the characteristics of several diagnostic groups (i.e. defective delinquent, sociopathic personality, antisocial or asocial retardate, emotionally disturbed, pseudopsychopath). Therefore, in place of a restrictive label, we offered the following behavioral descriptions:

1. Handles problems with peers and staff by acting out physically.

2. Continually blames others for difficulties she encounters.
3. Responds defiantly to authority figures.
4. Interest and involvement in program activities is negative and hostile.
5. Responds in a hostile manner to instruction and constructive criticism.
6. Openly rejects staff attempts to deal with problems.
7. Has difficulty accepting limits which are placed on her behavior.
8. Manipulative behavior is detrimental to her own and peers' adjustment.

Each of these individuals displayed a primitive level of social functioning, was action oriented, and possessed a limited self-concept. They ranged in age from 15 to 22 (3 residents were between 27 to 31) and functioned in the mild and borderline categories of measured intellectual potential (65-80 on Wechsler Intelligence Tests). The majority were characterized as cultural-familial retardates.

Prior to the establishment of the readjustment unit, individuals who exhibited the aforementioned behavior were excluded from the program because of their inability or unwillingness to participate. In most instances, these individuals were handled in a highly punitive and untherapeutic manner. Because of their disruptive and aggressive behavior, these residents would spend long periods of time in seclusion away from the general population. The possibility of such an individual returning to the community was nil, in that they were not permitted to participate in the institution's rehabilitative programs. This method of treatment not only increased and encouraged hostility and aggressiveness toward the institution and its staff, but totally ignored the worth, dignity, and needs of the individual.

The establishment of the readjustment unit enabled the institution to dispense with many of its punitive forms of treatment and to approach each individual as a unique human being. Based on a foundation of individual and small group dynamics, staff was encouraged to approach situations and behavior in a preventive rather than punitive manner. Prevention, responsibility, and appropriate social interactions became the guidelines to treatment.

Institutional routine was replaced by individualized concern. Antiseptic cleaning of the building gave way to antiseptic and preventive intervention in situations before they reached a crisis level. Responsibility rather than institutionalized dependency was encouraged. Staff was continually utilized to enhance appropriate and rewarding social interactions among residents.

In the two years from July, 1967 to July, 1969, a total of thirty-nine students moved through the readjustment unit. Sixteen were discharged from the institution; two were on leave of absence; two were transferred to our psychiatric unit; five more appropriately placed in our behavior modification unit; and twelve were functioning more appropriately in the general institutional population. Two were transferred to a less desirable setting. So as not to be misleading, the census of the cottage was thirty-six prior to the establishment of the revised program in July of 1967. The capacity in December 1968 was twenty-four. Many of those transferred had been inappropriately placed in the unit.

The program within the readjustment unit evolved in four distinct stages each based on our experiences. Stage one of program development was the outgrowth of an emergency situation, and therefore, planning and availability of resources were minimal. The program developed after the unit was locked and populated with thirty-six residents. The attendant staff was selected on the basis of supervisor recommendations and their past work performance. Professional involvement and support was inconsistent. No formalized in-service training program was initiated for the staff. This stood out as the most glaring oversight in the entire experience.

The major objectives were to cut down on the number of aggressive and disruptive incidents and to attempt to help these individuals progress through the institution. A step-by-step progression was established, based on an individual's behavior within the cottage. Those who behaved appropriately (conformed to expected standards) could be returned to the general institutional population. The ideal progression called for an increase in a student's activities and programs outside the unit with each month of appropriate behavior. The first month of a student's program was limited to cottage activities (i.e. occupational therapy, recreation, social activities, movies, individual counseling). During the second month a student could begin a half-day academic or vocational assignment outside the cottage. This could be increased to a full day's activities in the third month. With continued appropriate behavior, a student was eligible to participate in evening and weekend recreational activities during her fourth month of residence. Discharge from the unit could be obtained under ideal circumstances in a five-month period. This ideal was never approached, with the average length of stay during the first twenty-one months of the program being ten and one-half months for those discharged and twenty-one months for those still in residence. The program itself met a great deal of resistance from various members of the cottage team and institutional staff. They viewed the locking of the cottage as a return to the dark ages (prior to 1955 all cottages were locked). In part, this accounted for the following statement by a staff psychologist, which summarized the experiences during stage one: "The program worked for some, it may have harmed others, and for others it had no effect at all."

Evaluation, a clarification of goals, a definition of population to be served, and staff development accompanied stage two. The behavioral descriptions which have previously been mentioned were established. The population was reduced from thirty-six to twenty-four. The population reduction was accomplished by attempting to define each individual's difficulty and finding the most appropriate placement. With a smaller resident population and more clearly defined goals, each individual was treated as such and our focus changed from control to prevention. The preventive approach brought cries of favoritism and unfairness from the students but enabled us to move away from the punitive aspects of the program (medication and seclusion). In turn, we no longer had to deal with the guilt feelings which were activated each time an upset occurred. We returned to each girl her right to think and to be an individual, and in turn we expected her to accept reasonable responsibilities. Consequences of actions were clarified and destructive and aggressive behavior were no longer accepted. The students, as individuals and as a group, were expected to govern their actions. We maintained the previously established criteria for progression with only minor alterations. A variety of methods was utilized to assist staff in their daily functioning (films, discussions, formal and informal classes, supervision, on-the-spot consultation, and support from staff throughout the institution).

Stage three was ushered in with a physical change in cottage setting. We moved into a smaller unit whose physical arrangements and facilities were more appropriate to our needs. We continued our emphasis on prevention and responsibility. The majority of our students possessed the work skills necessary for job placement. However, we became increasingly aware that the real problem rested in our students' inability to function in interpersonal relationships and situations. They continually demonstrated a lack of concern for themselves and others. Coercion and homosexuality were most often the basis of relationships. We altered our method of approach to center around the small group where these difficulties might most appropriately be handled. Additionally, having a semi-locked unit (a majority of students left the cottage for academic or vocational assignments) created numerous difficulties. Lines of communication were not well established and inappropriate behavior was being sanctioned and reinforced. The majority of the institution staff were terrified by our students, and therefore, were hesitant to set or enforce limits. This predicament as well as a careful examination of our own feelings regarding keeping our students totally separate from the general institution led to stage four, our present program.

CURRENT PROGRAM

The current program is the culmination of our successful and not so successful experiences in learning to work with and understand the needs and demands of this type of individual. Basic to the functioning of the program is the belief that social skills and behavioral control can best be learned in a small group situation where structured social interaction and confrontations can take place.

The program is divided into two parts. The first part entails participation and involvement in the following types of structured activities: academic school, occupational therapy; recreation; individual counseling, group therapy, and assorted supervised institutional activities (i.e. cleaning, laundry, ironing, serving meals, homework periods, leisure time activities). Special emphasis is placed on prevention, emotional control, and responsible behavior. All of the activities are geared to here and now situations and relationships as well as to a clarification of past experiences and misunderstandings. A number of new experiences are provided in which the individual can begin to succeed and to view herself as a productive and capable individual. Such activities include making and altering personal clothing, making sandals and jewelry, ceramics, skits, talent shows, puppet theater, and student government. Through continued structured interactions students become attuned to the needs and difficulties of their peers, and are given the opportunity to give and share as well as to receive. Students suggested and carried through on a project to make Christmas toys for children at Pennhurst State School and Hospital, and have undertaken a Christmas wreath project through which funds were raised to purchase additional craft supplies for the unit. Each individual is encouraged and given a wide range of opportunities to develop basic communicative skills. In this way they are able to communicate in meaningful and appropriate ways their needs, feelings, and desires. Hopefully students will no longer find it necessary to communicate by acting out.

The second part of the program entails participation and residence in a small "social living unit." This unit is an attempt to establish a homelike environment which will better prepare students for return to the community. Emphasis is placed on meaningful social interactions and relationships, self-help skills, homemaking (housekeeping, menu planning, shopping, budgeting, preparation of meals), vocational attitudes and community experiences. Students share responsibility for the functioning of the kitchen. A small grocery store within the unit is utilized for learning to shop, budget, and use money. Students are given the opportunity to learn to comfortably operate a variety of household appliances. Trips into the community for social and cultural events are made possible by utilizing volunteers from Bucknell University and Pennsylvania State University. Excursions are planned to local factories, workshops, stores, banks, and employment agencies when possible. Students earn money for trips and personal items by washing cars, picking berries, day work assignments, and selling craft projects. These students are also learning to tie fishing flies in a workshop situation. Income received from this project will be used to help a student establish herself in the community when the program is completed. Although the majority of time in the "social living unit" is structured, specific periods of time remain unstructured. Students are expected to learn to occupy these periods with their own interests. In this way we hope that students might become accustomed to structuring their leisure time in the community with constructive activities.

The cottage population is divided into four groups of six students each. The division is based on the degree of displayed aggressiveness and involvement in the current program. Every attempt is made to separate complementary personality types. Each group is programmed as an independent unit within the cottage. Individuals are informed daily of their program involvement as well as the positive and negative aspects of their behavior through individual contacts, charts, and group meetings. Major emphasis is placed on the interpersonal and social aspects of each resident's behavior, and every attempt is made to involve students in all decisions regarding their program and future plans.

This program is made possible through an overall commitment of institutional resources and support. The unit is staffed by a full-time coordinator (social group worker), two part-time therapeutic activities workers, and a full-time teacher in addition to the regular child care staff. Several groups of volunteers from Bucknell University and Pennsylvania State University are utilized. Psychiatric consultation is provided by the superintendent.

The program as described appears workable, it appears to better meet the needs and demands of the population than previous approaches, and it is appealing to both students and staff. Definite changes have been observed in the attitudes, self-concepts, and daily functioning of individual residents.

However, the overall appearance of success is clouded by three issues. The first and most crucial issue is that of not having provided adequate training for unit staff during the early stages of program development. Superficial relationships and problems in communication between staff members tend to perpetuate and condone manipulative behavior. This in turn places unnecessary emotional pressures on staff and students and permits situations to develop which are anti-therapeutic. Shulman's[6] discussion of the game, "Who's On Top," accurately describes the type of difficulty encountered when lines of communication are inadequate and open to manipulation by students. Through a great deal of practice and success, residents have become skilled at dictating the reactions of staff and the terms for punishment or discipline. When staff became aware of how they were being used and refused to play the game by the established rules, an initially hostile reaction was encountered. Students became frustrated that their inappropriate needs were no longer being met and they were no longer in control. It was not until staff was able to share their newfound insights with the students that a new basis for relationships and interactions could develop. Each interaction between staff and students must be carefully analyzed in order to help staff understand their involvement in student's behavior, feelings, and reactions.[8] An intensive sensitivity training program is indicated.

Additional personnel to more adequately meet the needs and demands of this behaviorally disturbed group is also indicated. A 1:1 ratio of staff to student coverage is imperative if the full potential of this program and of each individual student is to be reached.

The third complicating factor involves the presence of certain personality constellations which present differential problems in treatment and management. The individual who used aggressive and acting out behavior as a defense against dealing with depression and the feelings of hopelessness and low self-esteem[3] will be approached differently than the individual who defends against schizophrenic thought processes by acting out.[4] These two groups of individuals can be treated within the established program with the assistance of chemotherapy. The third and largest clustering of individuals, those who fit Alexander's[2] and Aichhorn's[1] description of the "neurotic character disorder," present a major challenge. Each of these individuals functions under the faulty or fantasized premise that he is guilty of some untold (in many cases it is told) crime or act for which he must be punished. Success only reactivates the feelings of guilt; the cycle of sin, repentance, and failure perpetuates itself. Staff must be constantly aware and atuned to the meaning and desired payoff of such actions so as not to become an unknowing reinforcer in this maladaptive cycle. A total relearning and restructuring of perceptions and relationships must be built into each individual's program.

The treatment of all of these groups is further complicated by the induced dependency which institutions provide and the realistic fear of returning to a rejecting community. It is our belief that as the length of time spent in an institution increases for this type of individual, the probability of effecting change through treatment rapidly decreases. Early intervention and preventative action is strongly advocated as the prime treatment approach in dealing with the acting out retardate.[7]

We are still in our infancy and learning takes place every day. We are hopeful that our experiences and observations will lead to a better understanding of the problems all of us face in attempting to treat these long-forgotten individuals.

REFERENCES

1. Aichhorn, August: *Wayward Youth*. New York, Viking Press, 1965, pp. 167-186.
2. Alexander, Franz: *Fundamentals of Psychoanalysis*. New York, W. W. Norton Company, 1963, pp. 234-240.
3. Berman, Merrill J.: Mental retardation and depression. *Ment Retard*, 5:19-21, December, 1967.
4. Krinsky, Leonard W. and Jennings, Rose M.: The management and treatment of acting out adolescents in a separate unit. *Hosp Community Psychiatry*, 19(3):72-75, March, 1968.
5. Redl, Fritz and Wineman, David: *Controls From Within*. New York, The Free Press Paperback, 1965, 198-199.
6. Shulman, Lawrence: A game model theory of interpersonal strategies. *Social Work*, 13(3):16-22, July, 1968.
7. Weingold, Joseph T.: Towards a new concept of the delinquent defective. *Ment Retard*, 4(6):36-38, December, 1966.
8. Woloshin, Arthur A., Tardi, Guido, and Tobin, Arnold: De-institutionalization of mentally retarded men through use of a half-way house. *Ment Retard*, 4(3):21-25, June, 1966.

Chapter 9

CREATIVE ART EXPRESSION OF THE MENTALLY RETARDED

FLORENCE LUDINS-KATZ

THERE is a tremendous feeling of satisfaction in all people when they are able to express what they feel, whether it be great joy or great sorrow or just the experience of everyday living. To be able to dance and sing, to make music, to paint and sculpt is to come alive. The emotions pent up within us are released and take form in a meaningful way, meaningful to the creator and to the beholder.

It is a wonderful sensation to paint or sculpt and see the things you feel take shape before you—sometimes after great struggle, sometimes just a flowing and an outpouring. But how much more satisfying when others can share the experience with you, when art becomes a group activity, when there is an interchange and sharing with those working with you and with those who experience the finished work.

ART IN EDUCATION

In our present educational system, there is general acknowledgment of what art can do for the young child and every school program encourages children so that learning can be made more meaningful and enriched by their creativity and expressiveness. Sadly, as children grow older this natural outpouring is suppressed and either discontinued entirely or is made the handmaiden of other subjects such as reading or arithmetic. Creative

In this paper I will limit myself to painting and sculpture although what I have to say is equally true for all the arts. My experience is in teaching fine arts to both normal and mentally retarded persons of all ages, and thus I am confining my paper to my own personal experience.

art is not a learning experience for such specifics as "How many windows does a house have?" or "How do the leaves on a tree grow?" There is room for this kind of lesson, but call it observation and reinforcement, not art. Just at the time when children need so much to express their inner life, what they have to say and feel is crushed and becomes unimportant compared to facts they *must* learn. This is also true of the adult. Administrators often consider art as one of the "frills and fads" of education. But what is education if it is not encouraging the person to become vitally interested in all that goes on within him and around him, and to feel that he has something important to communicate—that he is an integral and living part of our culture—that he belongs?

Within each of us there is tremendous depth. When our feelings are bottled up, we dry up. When there is encouragement to express ourselves and when what we feel and think and say has an importance to others, we feel equal and competent and above all there is reason to be. We become important to ourselves and to society. We become a part of the scheme of things.

ART FOR THE MENTALLY RETARDED

But, you may ask, what has this to do with the mentally retarded? My answer is, everything. As great as is the importance of the expression of art to the normal, it is of much greater importance to the mentally retarded. Here we have a group of people who have the same feelings, the same desires, the same loves, the same hates, but who, through their intellectual inability, find it difficult to express themselves with words. In art often their feelings are able to come forth. It is like opening a closed box with unexpected depths. To be able to create a situation which encourages this emergence is the joy and the reward of teaching the mentally retarded.

The art program as described here is based on the premise that intelligence and emotion are not necessarily correlated—that a person of even very low intelligence may have an emotional drive to express himself and a desire to communicate with those around him. What he has to say is important to him and to us.

STEREOTYPES

Before describing the program I have set up for the mentally retarded I would like to challenge many of the stereotypes about
them. People ask, "Don't you find it dull and boring working with
the mentally retarded?" There is the assumption that the mentally retarded have nothing worthwhile to say. Since intellectually
they often cannot express themselves, they therefore are likewise
inadequate artistically. For many, art for the mentally retarded
consists of copying or of repetitive crafts. They believe that the
teacher should put a picture on the blackboard or a picture
should be given with the directions to copy exactly as possible.
They also believe that craft work should be laid out and the retarded person should put it together in a specified order without
any innovation or individuality, such as paint-by-number kits or
loom-weaving kits. In pottery, molds are used and wet clay is
merely poured, not formed or worked with. The student and the
teacher become bored and the results are, on the whole, use-
less and inadequate for any kind of growth. There is very little
real education taking place, although certain skills may be
learned.

Mentally retarded do have things to say even if they are intellectually unable to voice them. Feelings run very deep. Saying
what they feel may take many shapes.

> A woman of sixty who has never had a home of her own found
> delight in painting houses. This was what she wanted most—to have
> a home of her own. The houses were an infinite variety and color,
> but she always painted her dream, and we shared it with her.
> A young man in his thirties who was religious, painted many
> pictures of crosses in varying positions on varying backgrounds. This
> was his special devotion. Because he could not talk about it made
> his feelings and devotion no less ardent.
> Another young man in his thirties who loved to wander about the
> city, painted the University Campanile, subway stations, bridges,
> swimming pools. The world about him came to life with a double
> meaning when he could paint and show others his joy in what he
> saw.

But even more than specific things, so much of the work is an
imaginative outpouring of color, texture, and form. We find

among the mentally retarded the same variations in the things they paint or sculpt as we find in any group. The problem of the art teacher is to be careful not to be too directive and inhibit what the person wants to say and has to say—not to make the teacher's feeling so strong that the person painting will feel that he must comply and do what the teacher wishes.

Even though this is true of all teaching it is more basic in the teaching of the mentally retarded. These people have always been considered inadequate. They often try so much to please, that crushing their egos and making them conform to certain standards is not very difficult, although the standards are those of the teacher. Therefore, the teacher must be on guard not to allow himself to force his concepts on the mentally retarded, and to always remember that what they have to say is important to them and to us. He must be sensitive and aware of the first premise— the mentally retarded have something to say and they do have the ability to say it.

Another stereotype is that the mentally retarded have no power of concentration, that they can only scribble for a few minutes, then they are finished. Many feel there is nothing within them that will sustain a period of concentration. I have found in working with them that the concentration span varies as it will in any normal group. With stimulating color and materials, with no pressure, with encouragement and understanding, many can easily work for at least two hours, even refusing to take "breaks." This is by no means less than the ordinary attention span.

Very often work will be put away and continued the following week or weeks. The concept is not necessarily an immediate one. They will take the time and the effort to see the completion of what they wish to say as long as they feel it is important, and as long as the art teacher encourages the feeling that the statement being made is an important one.

Many believe that a mentally retarded person is constantly repetitive, that there is no room for growth, that changes do not occur. How false this is in the light of their production. There are some who for many weeks paint with only one color and even an experienced teacher will feel that this student has reached his limits. Suddenly he will burst forth in full color with a true feeling for spatial relationships. What a wonderful surprise for an art teacher to realize that his patience and encouragement made this possible. Then there are those who paint what they have learned—a formula in school, such as a house with a tree on either side. This student suddenly discovers that there are no restrictions, that he can paint what he feels, and the changes are so immediate and so far-reaching as to be exciting to all participating. There are those who are experimentalists and those who have found a formula, are comfortable in that formula, and tend to remain there. Others criticize their work, make changes, try to eliminate what they feel wrong, repeat what is satisfactory, making small changes as they go along. Others are satisfied and delighted with everything they produce. They are not alone. Look through the books on art and this tendency can be seen in many of our greatest artists. They tend to repeat what they feel is successful. This is how we can identify an artist's work even though we may have never seen this particular example. In art we call this "style." In the mentally retarded we often call it "repetition."

Another stereotype is that all mentally retarded people are alike, that since they cannot "think" they are all gay and childlike. Nothing could be further from the truth. Each is a complete individual with his own thoughts, feelings, likes, and dislikes. Their appearance and their personalities are totally different. One may be bright and sunny, another may be brooding and thoughtful, keeping his feelings within himself. Some make friends easily, others are loners. This difference in personality is immediately apparent in their art work. Some choose bright and sunny colors, others prefer the dark and somber hues. Some like to sculpt or draw large figures—the bigger the better, while others make miniatures and delight in the perfection of details. Their work is so different that in a whole roomful of art work, an experienced person can often pick out the work of each individual.

In working with art with the mentally retarded, let's put first things first. Although it is very important what the paintings do for us—the onlookers, the consumers—this is not the main issue. It is what the paintings do for the creator. To come into a room where the mentally retarded are painting or sculpting, to watch the faces, the concentration, the complete absorption, the animation, and the joy, is to know without question what the act of aesthetic production means to them. Here there is no rocking, no masturbation, no hesitancy, no vacant stare. Here each person is worthwhile in his own right. There are no feelings of inadequacy and inferiority.

QUALIFICATIONS FOR AN ART TEACHER

For those who would like to set up an art program, a few things must be borne clearly in mind. It is not necessary for the teacher to be an artist, but it is necessary for him to be an appreciator. He should be well versed in modern art and understand that expression is more important than representation. If the teacher is looking for exact reproduction, he may as well not begin. Failure and disappointment will be his lot and this will be quickly transferred to the students. They are sensitive to feelings, as are all students, and a great deal of harm can be done. This could add one more step to a feeling of failure and inadequacy on both the teacher's and the students' parts. The mentally retarded are already the lowest on the totem pole and their egos have suffered much. Do not add to this burden.

To be an inspiring teacher one must genuinely enjoy a free flow of form, color, and line. One must be able to stimulate and to appreciate what the students are doing and must understand the joy of creation at all levels. There is no room for falsehood or pussyfooting. The mentally retarded will easily spot any dishonesty. If the teacher genuinely enjoys and appreciates the true expression of his students' production, the art lesson will be a glowing example of adequacy and satisfaction.

Here expectations play a major role. If one truly expects that the students are capable of producing worthwhile art, the work will be exhilarating and fascinating both for the participants and for those who view the work. Something happens in the room. A teacher becomes a catalyst and indescribable results occur. I cannot understand the mechanism but when expectations are high, the students put forth a creative response and unforetold things just seem to happen spontaneously.

SETTING UP THE PROGRAM
Group Activity

In setting up a program, I use large tables with six or eight students around each table, sometimes seated, sometimes standing. Materials go in the center of the table. The student must find what he needs whether it is a particular color or material. He must learn to make choices of his own volition. Also art becomes a social experience, where each person can look at the other person's work and can be stimulated by it and enjoy it. Copying is never approved of. It is always accentuated that each person has something worthwhile to say—even if this is putting two colors together or two pieces of wood in an unusual or expressive way. When people are placed in corners by themselves at easels apart from the rest of the group, many anxieties set in. "Am I doing the right thing?" "What shall I paint?" "How shall I put this together?"

When people work around a table they feel their work is equal to anyone's. All share. They enjoy each other's work and are stimulated to produce in their own way. The other students will often make suggestions far superior and more acceptable than the teacher's. Only if the teacher can make each person proud of what he is doing, is he fulfilling his role. For instance, one in a group will start with lines. Soon others will try their hand at it, drawing lines, crossing lines, thick lines, thin lines, many lines, few lines, colored lines, and so forth. This is not copying but creating a stimulus to experiment. This is superior to a teacher saying, "Let's start with lines," or "What will many lines do?" If the teacher wishes, discussion can come later, with such questions as, "What did you feel when you were making these lines?" Never say, "This one is successful and this one is not successful." Negative comparisons are never made. Art is not a competitive sport. Each person who participates wins.

One of the most interesting lessons came about when one mentally retarded individual decided to use letters for his paintings. Since he did not know the alphabet, one of the other students showed him the letters on a piece of scrap paper.* Soon the

* When doing individual work one of the stipulations is that no one can work on another person's paper. This is the rule for the teacher as well.

second student began to make letters on his own page. The others around the table suddenly became interested and began to paint letters. The session became alive—all worked helping and teaching each other—laughing and joking. Each page began to look like a medieval manuscript or a page from the work of Sister Mary Corita. Some had large consecutive letters, some had small miscellaneous letters, some used many colors, some used few colors, but above all the students were animated and alive. The lesson came from within themselves. How different it would have been if the teacher had started by superimposing his will on the group, if he had said, "Now, let us all try to learn the alphabet, let us all work with letters."

Working around a large table stimulates group activity and very often all can share using a single piece of paper or board. But there are other times when a student wishes to work by himself. This provision can easily be made by setting up a second table nearby where others can work on their own ideas.

Materials

The materials in an art program should be stimulating, plentiful, inexpensive, and easy to use. Paints in a variety of colors should be in jars that will not tip over. (Baby food jars are excellent.) Plenty of glue, scraps of wood, cardboard, textured materials, colored papers and wool should be available. It is of the utmost importance in teaching (except when he is no longer an amateur) that the student must feel that the materials in themselves have little value. The value comes from within himself, from what he has created with the materials. Expensive leathers, costly woods, oil colors, make the teacher fearful of allowing students to experiment. The beauty of the material becomes the important thing, not the experience of creating.

I have seen classes in leather work where the teacher cuts the leather for fear of the student spoiling it, where the student is doled out a certain small piece of wood or metal. How can a student feel secure when the teacher is apprehensive of failure? In jewelry, cheap copper, white metal, brass—flat, round, square, thick, thin, not silver or gold, should be used. If a mistake is made such inexpensive materials can be put aside or redone or destroyed without feelings of guilt.

An excellent source of supplies is a hike with a large paper sack. In the city each student can collect wire, bits of metal, colored glass, wood, interesting nails, pieces of cardboard with unusual labels. In the country the hike with the paper sack results in small rocks, dried seed pods, bits of wood, bark, twigs. At the seashore there are shells, bits of driftwood, feathers, colored sands, grasses, water-worn objects. If each one collects what he finds most interesting, sculpture and collage can be made with only the cost of glue and nails. This can be made into a group project where all pool the materials or each can work with the things he himself has found and collected.

To illustrate a similar lesson, and there are innumerable examples, one of the boys came in to class full of excitement. A fence was being torn down and the old wood was so interesting. The teacher sent him out to bring in the wood. He looked at it and the teacher said, "What can you do with it?" He picked up a heavy piece of four by four and said, "This looks like a cross." "Well, then, make a cross." The next question was, "Are you satisfied?" "No," was the answer. "A Christ should be on it." "Make the Christ." The student went out and behind the school found a pile of junk from old cars. The bumper became the body, the carburetor became the head, pieces of wire became a crown of thorns, and, lo, a Christ was born!

Of course I do not mean to imply that there is no place for precious materials, but certainly not until the student is sure of himself and not until he has had sufficient experience and experimentation with inexpensive and found materials.

In a painting lesson it is much more important to have large cheap paper than small expensive sheets. However, the paper must be of a quality that the students do not feel frustrated because the paper falls apart when working on it. I would suggest rolls of heavy butcher paper or manilla. Tempera paint is cheap but the colors must be so stimulating and so varied that there is desire to paint. You cannot place ragged paper, dull and muddy colors on a table and expect people to have the urge to work. My criterion is that the colors must be interesting enough to make your mouth water. Brushes may be cheap but not so poor that the hair falls out and the brush lies limply on the paper. I would suggest a variety of sizes, 1 inch, ¾ inch, ½ inch, etc. The handles should be long enough and heavy enough so even those with motor disabilities can grasp them easily.

There are many places which are obsessed with cleanliness, where painting becomes a problem. Place large cheap plastic sheets on the tables so no one will be fearful of getting tables dirty. In this way there is also no problem of clean-up.

In a sculpture class, wood scraps may be obtained from a lumber yard or picture frame maker at no cost and can be stimulating. Students will sit for hours gluing and nailing—sometimes trying to reproduce cars and houses and at other times creating just for the fun of the shapes and sizes growing before their eyes. A good coat of tempera paint will add much to the effect.

SUMMARY

As an artist and as a teacher I know that the art of the mentally retarded can be exhilarating and rewarding to the teacher, to the retarded, and to the general public.

To the teacher there is the feeling that through his understanding and stimulation something wondrous has been born—a work of art.

To the retarded, he can be equal to all. He is adequate, no longer a failure. He is able to share his feelings, his thoughts, his hopes, and his sorrows. He can enjoy what he produces and others can enjoy it with him.

To the general public there is an enrichment. Many of the works produced stand as art in their own right. The vigor, the use of color, the organization, and the intensity of feeling are a worthwhile contribution to our society.

Chapter 10

ROLE OF THE PHYSICIAN

PETER COHEN

THE physician who first suspects the presence of mental retardation or who subsequently confirms the diagnosis is in a vital position to provide appropriate information and counseling for parents. He can assist them in developing healthier attitudes in regard to the problem and minimize the emotional impact on them and, in turn, on their affected child.

In interpretation of the nature of the retardation and counseling of the parents, the physician must be sympathetic toward the retarded child and forbearing toward the parents. Many parents resent the physician who informs them bluntly, sometimes with too little examination or investigation, that their child is retarded and nothing can be done. When the phrase, "he will never be any better" is used, the physician means that the relationship between the mental and chronological age will remain constant during the developmental period. The parents, however, interpret this to mean that the child will make no intellectual progress whatever and they become even more discouraged. Later, when the child shows signs of progress, the parents begin to feel that the doctor was wrong in his prognosis and nurture the hope that the child will begin to develop normally. This produces a lack of confidence and trust in the physician because of his own earlier hasty interpretation.

The physician who evaluates the child must recognize that, although some parents realize the slowness of the child at the moment, they consider this to be temporary. By a process of rationalization, they relate it to some vague cause and expect that the child will be normal eventually. It is the physician's responsibility to project the child's development into the future to the

144

best of his ability, so that the parents can plan realistically and have no false illusions or expectations. Institutionalization may be one of the alternatives to be considered in the future management of the child, but the physician should assist the parents to make that decision rather than to make it for them.

A series of office visits may be necessary to answer the many other questions of the parents. For this, the physician should adopt an "open door" policy for anything that pertains to the progress of the child and his physical needs. He will continue to be of vital importance to the family of a retarded child long after the diagnosis is established and the immediate needs are satisfied. Crises will occur inevitably, and he must be ready to help the parents with them.

Plans for school will have to be made after the diagnosis has been established. Parents will raise questions about sibling relationships, whether the normal child or children in the family will be affected by having a retarded child at home, whether the parents should have more children, or whether the siblings have a greater risk of having similarly affected children. Honest answers can be of value in avoiding the emotional crises in the family that may affect not only the retarded child but the normal children as well.

COMMUNITY RESOURCES

Many physicians have only one solution for the retarded, particularly the moderately or severely retarded, and that is institutionalization. They need to be aware of the many community facilities that are available and therefore to explore every possible approach that may increase the retarded child's chances for positive adaptation.[1] Now, only 4 per cent of the retarded population live in institutions, the others live out their lives in the community. This requires an array of community facilities to provide the necessary services. There is an increasing emphasis on having the retarded child live within his family, where he can receive stimulus, care, love, and encouragement to realize more of his potential.

There are wide ranges of services available in many communities. They are available from a variety of professions and organizations that assist in the care of retarded individuals during their lifetime. These can be very beneficial in assisting the parents to cope with the problems of retardation.

A homemaker can assist the mother with her family chores when the care of the affected child becomes a burden beyond her physical and emotional endurance, or baby sitting services may give the mother an opportunity to satisfy her personal needs. A plan of respite care can be developed for those family crises which inevitably develop. These "respite" services provide care for the affected individual when he cannot be cared for by his mother because of her own illness, a new pregnancy, other illness emergency in the family, or death of a relative which takes the mother away from home. This service also permits the rest of the family to enjoy themselves together at the time of a family vacation without the extra care of the retarded individual.

A day nursery can provide enrichment for the toddler-aged child and also serve as a meeting place for the mother with others who have similarly affected children. Appropriate treatment can be instituted there and continued more adequately for the child with such associated defects as cerebral palsy, hearing defects, or epilepsy. At school age, the child will enter a class most suited to his ability—either one for the educable retarded or the trainable retarded. However, some children may be so severely handicapped that it would be unrealistic to enroll them in such classes; for them, a day care program can provide necessary supervision and sensory stimulation.

Adolescents and young adults should have educational counseling, personal adjustment training, or occupational training which might lead to competitive employment. Sheltered workshops can provide training and work opportunities adapted to the skills of the retarded individual. Adequate resources for recreation should be available, some may even fit into such organized activities as scouting or camping. Religious education should be provided within the family unit.

Sometimes, even the question of marriage will be raised, when an appropriate mate is found. If marriage does take place, the questions of childbearing, birth control, or sterilization will arise.

As the retarded individual grows older, guardianship plans

must be developed for the time when his parents are no longer available to supervise him. Boarding homes can provide an opportunity for continued social supervision. In addition to survivor's insurance and old age assistance benefits, "aid to the totally disabled" benefits provide for his needs and make it possible for him to remain in the community.

For some of the retarded, out of home placement may be necessary. This will include those whose families cannot accept the child in the home in spite of efforts at counseling. Under such circumstances the child will suffer greater emotional trauma by remaining in his own home than by being placed in a residential facility appropriate to his needs. Some parents who are no longer able to provide a home, may have to place the child in a family care home where foster parents can continue to provide the necessary supervision and guidance. A residential school may be required for the individual who cannot receive an adequate educational program in his own community.

Public health nurses can direct parents to appropriate follow-up programs. For example, children who require special diets can be controlled more adequately by the visit of a nurse who knows the family and has the help of a nutritionist. She can also assist the parents in recognizing the child's developmental levels, and suggest to them ways to assist him in developing more social competence.

Family agencies, both denominational and nondenominational can be helpful in counseling. In most communities, organized parent groups provide great emotional support and an outlet for shared experience. Also, for the severely retarded with multiple handicaps, long-time residential care under public or private auspices may be the best program.

In addition to the many community services enumerated, which provide specific programs for the retarded and supportive counseling for the family, there is a need for a multiple therapeutic approach which includes psychiatric services, supportive play therapy, behavior modification, and psychotropic medications.

The State of California has taken a significant and innovative step in providing a community resource whereby the mentally retarded and their families can be assisted in obtaining services appropriate to their needs. In 1965, a bill[10] was passed to initiate the development of a network of regional centers to provide an array of services which include diagnosis, counseling, and funds for financing programs in or out of the home, for the welfare of the retarded individual. The purpose of the legislation was to insure that all individuals who were recognized as being retarded would have alternatives to state hospital care. It also shifted the responsibility of the state from the time the retarded individual enters a state hospital to the time when he is diagnosed as needing "specialized care." Heretofore, families were unable to take advantage of the many available services for the retarded because of lack of funds. Now, when a physician recognizes the need of a specific service for a patient under his care, he can enlist the cooperation of the regional center to plan with him and the family the way in which the service might be provided and funded.

Counseling, a major activity of the program, is provided by social workers, as well as public health nurses, nutritionists, and physicians. The counselor assigned to the family is required to review periodically with the parents the status of the retarded individual and the program in which he is involved, whether in his own home or in a residential facility. The counselor is also available for crisis intervention to aid the retarded individual and his family in many ways. He becomes an ombudsman to cut through the bureaucratic rules and regulations that sometimes impede and frustrate everyone—the retarded individual, his family, and the professional workers. The counselors and the other members of the professional staff are aware of the variety of programs available in the community and throughout the state which might be beneficial to the retarded individual and thereby protect him from the frustrations of inadequate services and care which might influence his emotional development.

This kind of intervention may help the retarded individual develop to his maximum potential without the emotional overlay that can occur when parents are frustrated and emotionally upset in regard to the status of their child. Experience has indicated that, for many parents as well as for the retarded child, this program has been extremely successful. Parents are relieved when they realize their child is in an appropriate program and there is an agency whose representatives will continue to be concerned with his needs, even when they are no longer available to provide protection and supervision. Lifetime supervision by the Regional Center is available through a guardianship plan.

THE MENTALLY RETARDED PATIENT

Mental retardation is the manifestation of a variety of conditions due to many causes. Some are associated with biochemical disorders of genetic determination, which include such inborn errors of metabolism as those resulting from deficient or missing enzymes. Other genetic implications include microcephaly or tuberous sclerosis; still others are associated with a variety of chromosomal abnormalities, of which Down's syndrome is the most frequent. Some can result from insult during the prenatal period, such as infection, or such perinatal factors as anoxia or birth injury. Hemolytic disease of the newborn also carries with it a high risk of damage to the central nervous system, and prematurity predisposes to brain damage and, therefore, to mental retardation.

A variety of other handicapping conditions may be associated with mental retardation, including visual and hearing loss of varying degrees, convulsive states, such physical handicapping conditions as cerebral palsy and, sometimes, emotional problems superimposed upon the intellectual and physical involvement. The functioning of the retarded individual, therefore, is influenced by the many associated conditions that may be present as well as by the degree of intellectual development.

Mental retardation manifests itself in varying degrees, from the most profound in which the individual is completely dependent on others for every need, to the very mildest form which may not be recognized, in which the person may not be considered much different from his neighbors and can merge into the community and be employed.

The fact that a child is different can have a profound effect on the parents' emotional state which, in turn, may influence the child's behavior and response to training and education. This superimposed influence can affect the emotional well-being of the child and interfere further with his ability to attain whatever his basic potential might be with otherwise appropriate training. All parents, in anticipating the birth of a child, hope to have one to whom they can point with pride, who can be compared with the children of their relatives and friends, and about whose accomplishments they can be proud as he grows and develops. The number of cameras and the volume of film sold attest to the importance placed in having a child to show off as handsome and intelligent.

Therefore, the realization that a child is different, not particularly attractive and obviously retarded intellectually, comes as a great shock and disappointment. This can result in various reactions. Parents may hope that the apparent retardation is only temporary and that, when the cause is determined, a treatment program will permit the child to "catch up." After appropriate evaluation, when they finally realize that their child is not going to be normal and will continue to function less adequately than his peers, some parents develop guilt feelings. Since the child is part of their own germ plasm and they are responsible for the child's conception, it seems to them that one or the other must be solely responsible for the child's defects. Sometimes these guilt feelings result in projection of the blame onto someone else, e.g. onto the doctor who delivered the child. It is necessary and important for the physician who evaluates the child to give the parents an opportunity to vent any guilt feelings or projection onto others. Clarification of these feelings will have a beneficial effect on the milieu in which the child is raised.

As their retarded child grows older, the parents may react to the burden of care by an unconscious wish to be rid of their problem; this often results in overcompensation in the form of excessive care, protection, and concern. Sometimes, when their demands for the needs of the child are not met, they develop bitter hostility towards relatives, doctors, neighbors, school, or community in general. Such attitudes can have a deleterious effect on the child and influence his behavior and attainments so that he becomes even more inadequate in social behavior and overall functioning. As a result, the child may become autistic, develop increased tension, become hyperactive or poorly motivated.[2, 7, 8]

EMOTIONAL REACTIONS OF THE
MENTALLY RETARDED

Menolascino[7] reported a study of 616 children at the Nebraska Psychiatric Institute, 191 of whom displayed prominent psychiatric problems with and without associated mental retardation. The frequency of emotional disturbances tended to increase sharply in children four years of age and over and twice as many boys displayed psychiatric problems. There is a two-fold increase in the frequency of emotional disturbances in the mentally retarded children when compared with those under eight in the general child population (in which an incidence of 10 per cent has been reported).[7, 11] One hundred and fifty-one of the group were both emotionally disturbed and mentally retarded.

There are conflicting opinions concerning the vulnerability of the mentally retarded to general pressure reactions. Gardner[3] could not find any epidemiological data which would shed any light on the question of depressive reactions in the mentally retarded. The reports he cited indicated that the rate of occurrence among the retarded was lower than that in the general population. However, he did note that the mentally retarded are highly susceptible to serious behavioral disturbances, sometimes with evidence of schizophrenic reactions which might be in excess of those found in the general population, as well as a high incidence of psychotic episodes of excitement.

Patients with mild to moderate degrees of mental retardation often recognize their inadequacy and the overt or covert rejection by peers or older people. These feelings of inadequacy, helplessness, and rejection may find their expression in overt symptoms of depression, according to Glaser,[4] and very often produce anger against the environment, especially when superiority of siblings, schoolmates, and friends is obvious. This anger is then expressed in acting-out behavior which may be directed against those who control the retarded child, which may lead to further restrictions and more severe control and punishment by the parents. From these feelings of helplessness and anger, because of fear of punishment or inability to effectively show hostility toward the controlling persons, the retarded individual may direct his anger toward younger children, defenseless individuals, animals, or inanimate objects.

INFLUENCE OF THE RETARDED ON PARENTS AND SIBLINGS

It must be remembered that the retarded individual is part of a family group. His limitations affect not only the parents but also the siblings.[8] Cummings, *et al.*[2] and Philips[9] have detailed the common emotional reactions of the parents of the retarded. These reactions consist of anxiety and depression, which manifest themselves as withdrawal, guilt, oversolicitude, resentment, and hostility. Recognition of these feelings may be important in the appropriate resolution of the problem faced by the retarded child, can result in decrease of social function and maternal caretaking competence and, in turn, can develop into alienation of parent from child, parent from parent, and parent from surrounding social groups.

How the siblings are affected has not been clearly documented. Kaplan[5] points out that families with retarded children must be helped to cope with the problems in a way that enhances rather than constricts or distorts the growth of all family members. In her work with siblings she found a surprising lack of awareness of families and professionals of the siblings' role in the family's attempt at coping with the retardation. At the New Haven Regional Center she accumulated evidence to suggest that siblings of retarded children are often adversely affected. She organized a discussion group of adolescent siblings of retarded children to try to learn more about the attitudes of siblings and the effects of the retarded child on them. From this, she found several factors to be important, e.g. the way the family talks about the retardation, how they deal with their own aggression toward the retarded child, how they teach the normal child to do this, how they handle the community relationships with the retarded family member, and how they assist their normal children in understanding and explaining the issues involved.

Cummings, *et al.*[2] have very aptly pointed out that parental caretaking competence is the most important single manpower resource available. Therefore, a means must be found to help prevent the parents of retarded children from developing personality features which curtail their ability to offer a psychological climate which is conducive to their optimal ego development. Maintenance of the parent's self-esteem and confidence in their ability to care adequately for their children is of benefit not only to the parents of deficient children but to their other offspring as well.

SUMMARY

The mentally retarded individual suffers from a condition which is influenced by many factors, not the least of which is the attitude of his parents and those close to him. His physician is of importance to him and his family in establishing the cause and degree of retardation and to reevaluate the needs of the retarded individual with time and any change of circumstance. The retarded individual's eventual place in society will be determined by the degree of retardation, the opportunities for counseling, and the availability of community programs which are appropriate to his needs. His emotional impact on his family and, in turn on him, can be ameliorated by the use of these opportunities in a constructive way.

REFERENCES

1. Chess, S. and Korn, S.: Temperament and behavior disorders in mentally retarded children. *Arch Psychiatr*, 23:122-130, 1970.
2. Cummings, S. T., Bailey, H. C., and Rie, H. E.: Effects of the child's deficiency on the mother: A study of mothers of mentally retarded, chronically ill and neurotic children. *Am J Orthopsychiatr*, 36:595-608, 1966.
3. Gardner, W. I.: Occurrence of severe depressive reactions in the mentally retarded. *Am J Psychiatr*, 124:386-388, 1967.
4. Glaser, K.: Masked depression in children and adolescents. *Am J Psychother*, 21:565-574, 1967.
5. Kaplan, F.: Siblings of the Retarded. In Sarason, S. B., and Doris, J. L. (Eds.): *Psychological Problems in Mental Deficiency*. New York, Harper and Row, 1969 (4th ed.).
6. Krug, O.: *Career Training in Child Psychiatry*. Washington, D.C., American Psychiatric Association, 1964, pp. 37-45.
7. Menolascino, F. J.: Psychiatric aspects of mental retardation in children under eight. *Am J Orthopsychiatr*, 35:852-861, 1965.
8. Michaels, J. and Schucman, H.: Observations on the psychodynamics

of parents of retarded children. *Am J Ment Defic,* 66:568-573, 1962.

9. Philips, I.: Psychopathology and mental retardation. *Am J Psychiatr,* 124:27, 1965.

10. State of California: *Assembly Bill 225.* Sacramento, California State Assembly, 1969.

11. Werkman, S. L.: Childhood Emotional Disorders. In Deutsch, H., and Fishman, H. (Eds.): *Encyclopedia of Mental Health.* New York, F. Watts, Inc., 1963, pp. 302-312.

Chapter 11

PARENTS AND SIBLINGS OF THE RETARDED

Ernest F. Pecci

INTRODUCTION

IT is difficult to understand the full impact of a handicapped child upon a family. First we must have some understanding of the impact of a healthy child upon the lives of his parents and siblings—the meaning of parenthood, the expectations and goals of each parent, the joy of giving, of sharing, of watching and reexperiencing the mystery of life unfold before their eyes, and the feeling that comes with knowing they are part of it. But what of the anxieties, the self-doubts, the disappointments, the loss of patience, the exasperations, the constant drain of energy and emotions? The raising of a healthy child puts a demand for stability and maturity upon each parent, the need for economic security, a family structure based upon mutual respect, easy communication, and clear guidelines for decision making, as well as the assistance of the outer greater society with its time-honored institutions, churches, medical, and recreational facilities to help the growing child along the developmental milestones to that day when he, too, can become an independent contributor to the society in which he lives.

And what of the child who is born "different," whose intellectual and physical handicaps delay or prevent his smooth transition along the developmental chain to maturity and independence? A child where the usual guidelines and supportive services to integrate him into society are lacking?

The handicapped child is not only physically or mentally disadvantaged, but socially excluded, physically deprived of the opportunities for exploration and the new experiences open to his siblings, and high risk for an unnatural and often pathologic

155

mother-child relationship which could further increase his inhibition, dependency, and disturbed self-concept. This is an attempt to clarify some of the complex factors modifying the impact of the retarded child upon his family, along with implication for therapeutic intervention.

EFFECTS OF THE RETARDED CHILD UPON FAMILY AUTONOMY

Only recently has society shown some willingness to consider alternatives to the isolated residential institution for its atypical or deviant children. The growth, in the past decade, of day care centers, special schools, developmental clinics, sheltered workshops, and activity programs for multiply handicapped children has eased the burden of care sufficiently to encourage parents to keep their retarded child within the home. Gradually, overwhelming evidence is being accumulated which shows that even severely retarded children can obtain considerable benefit from remaining in a warm and accepting family environment in contrast to their counterparts who are placed in institutions at an early age. They tend to be more sociable, more acceptable in behavior and appearance, and more independent in self-help skills. However, the family needs help in integrating a handicapped child into its social structure, and unless feelings about the handicapped child are understood, the entire family may become handicapped around his care.

Every member of a family modifies directly or indirectly all of the many interactional patterns within the family. The retarded child, too, is capable of both changing his environment and modifying behavioral responses toward him. To understand the nature of this influence, we must be able to visualize the family unit as a dynamically functioning system with personally and socially motivated goals and expectations of performance for each member. Ideally it functions as an integrated unit to cope with the anticipated developmental crisis of each child as he progresses through a natural cycle from birth to maturity, and each member is generally defined or treated according to his particular role at each stage of this cycle (i.e. baby, toddler, first grader, college student, teacher, mother, etc.). In the process, both parents must engage in much experimentation and make many decisions of a trial-and-error nature with an eye toward future expectations. Meanwhile they can obtain some feedback as to how well they are succeeding by comparing their child with other children of the same age. All the while the child's progress or lack of it is a continual reflection of credit or blame to the parents.

Every delay, especially in the commonly compared areas of walking, talking, height, and weight, is a source of mild to progressive anxiety on the part of the parents. But the real crisis occurs only at the point where the diagnosis of "mental retardation" is made by the physician and *accepted* by the parents. Here, the entire value system of the parents (based upon the value system of their society), that worth is commensurate with expected capabilities, must undergo a vital change. Either that, or they must reject the child who had been up to now an object of love and a source of high future expectations.

Farber[2] described how parents suffer what he terms "career frustration" at the point of realization that their child is mentally retarded. This is usually followed by a period of depression often expressed as "living in a void," or "there's nothing to live for now." All of the family members must reorient their lives with respect to the retarded child. The search begins for services, advice, and support. The usual pattern is for the child's pediatrician to refer the family to one of the large diagnostic clinics which are now cropping up in all of the major cities. Here the child undergoes extensive physical, neurological, and psychological examinations, expensive laboratory procedures such as electroencephalogram and pneumoencephalograms, and has blood and urine samples submitted to a variety of tests including chromosome studies. However, whatever hopes or expectations the parents may have had from all this expenditure of professional time and energy is usually very short-lived. The child is usually given a vague or meaningless diagnosis which tends to only further alienate the parents from their child, and is then referred back to the referring pediatrician who is not greatly helped by this new label and who is unequipped to handle the child and parents' attendant problems within a busy of-

fice practice and outside the fringe of his general specialty. It is not unusual for parents to be told of their child's handicap in a manner which intensifies their distress, leaving their major questions unanswered, or else given explanations which leave them feeling misinformed and no less confused than before.*
They receive diagnostic labels rather than reasonable answers to their very basic questions which they must have before they can make important decisions regarding the needed change in family thinking and structure to help integrate the handicapped child:

1. What is the cause of our child's retardation?
2. Have we personally contributed to his condition?
3. Is the condition hereditary?
4. How shall we explain him to our children, friends, neighbors?
5. Will our child ever walk, talk, attend school, be independent?
6. Is there a drug or operation that might make him brighter?
7. What will be his effect on our other children?
8. What will happen to him after we are gone?

Parents need constructive answers to these questions in order to prepare themselves psychologically and emotionally for the stresses ahead and to make realistic decisions based upon their existing economic and physical resources. Future planning is impossible without some estimation of the life expectancy and the ultimate level their retarded child will be able to attain in the areas of social adaptability and independent living. Lacking appropriate answers to their basic questions, parents tend to proceed on a confused day-to-day basis trying to cope piecemeal with each crisis as it occurs while developing pathologic defenses to help them to weather a turbulent sea of inner anxiety and

* In reviewing more than a hundred such reports from the best diagnostic clinics in this area, I would judge that over 90 percent of the final diagnoses can be summarized as follows: "Chronic brain syndrome probably related to intra-uterine cerebral anoxia or perinatal causes of unknown etiology with associated moderate to severe mental retardation." Of the remaining 10 per cent most of the specific diagnoses such as Down's syndrome were already made or suspected by the referring pediatrician.

periodic swells of desperation. A retarded child appearing early in the marriage of a young couple may have an especially deleterious effect on the family by curtailing the desire of the parents to further increase the family size, by severely restricting the family's recreational and social activities, and causing a general family withdrawal from community life.

REALITY STRESSES UPON THE MOTHER AS PRIMARY CARETAKER

The raising of a healthy or "normal" child in our complex society is an arduous task requiring optimal communication and mutual support between the parents as well as a variety of skills which, unfortunately, are usually learned through the process of experimentation. Little wonder that new parents feel very inadequate in their mothering and parenting roles. The young mother of a first-born retarded child is especially unprepared for her responsibilities. With no previous experience or adequate basis for comparisons she must cope with a variety of roles thrust upon her by necessity and by the expectations of our society.

Diagnostician

In our society the early care of the child is left largely in the hands of the mother who is constantly faced with a variety of minor emergencies to which she must respond with some kind of decision. When her child has a slight fever, or has a fall, or cuts his finger should she immediately consult the family physician, or is it safe to wait? Gradually the older parents learn to develop an optimistic or philosophic attitude based upon repeated reassurances by their pediatrician that their child has not suffered a brain concussion, or eaten something poisonous, or is going to get blood poisoning, that a poor appetite may be normal, that he will get over his rash in a couple of days, and that his diarrhea is "something which is going around now." But what of the parent of the severely retarded child who is highly susceptible to respiratory and ear infections, allergies and digestive problems, frequently whimpers as if in pain, has difficulty chewing and swallowing food, has severe orthopedic problems or congenital heart disease and is subject to a variety of epileptic-type seizures? How are they to interpret a new emergency and where should they take their child for help? Private physicians are ill-equipped to handle chronic medical conditions which are outside the usual problems of their practice. Although they can offer the parents support, they must be less optimistic as to the prognosis of the various presenting symptoms. Mothers of retarded children often continue to maintain a hyperresponse to every gasp or cry, and many live in constant fear that their child will die while unattended.

Psychologist

Parents are imbued with the awesome responsibility of developing the personalities and instilling a sense of identity in their children through their actions and attitudes of acceptance or rejection. The "mother-child" bond normally begins at birth.* Mothering behavior is now known to be a primarily learned, rather than instinctual, process elicited by various instructional responses from the baby such as smiling, clinging, sucking, and crying. However, the handicapped child often lacks the ability to stimulate his mother's normal maternal responses. On the contrary, his lethargy, irritability, inability to suck properly or swallow food instills anxiety, frustration and even disgust upon the part of the mother who, in turn, projects her own state of tension and insecurity back upon the child. This pattern may result in a cycle whereby the child gradually becomes less affectionate, more apathetic or negativistic, and lacking in normal motivation for social contact. Sometimes the mother is confused as to the cause or reason for certain negative behavior. It becomes increasingly more difficult for her to differentiate between the negative behavioral reactions which she is inadvertently developing through her inexperienced handling of her child and those reac-

---

* Dr. Lester Sontag, Director of the Fels Research Institute for the Study of Human Development, Antioch College, Ohio, has compiled a volume of evidence pointing to the fact that the mother-child bond actually begins in the womb: "The fetus reacts to sound, to his mother's smoking, to her grief, fear, anxiety, discomfort, and fatigue, and is presumably molded by these experiences." We might speculate as to whether this might be a reason for the very high incidence of birth defects and "minimal brain damage" in adopted children.

tions which are common to a greater or lesser extent in all children suffering from brain damage at birth, such as immaturity, hyperactivity, irritability, poor impulse control, low tolerance for frustration, unpredictable temper tantrums, and exaggerated fear reactions.

New crises occur in adolescence as the child's growing size, sexual development, and increasing awareness that he is "different" makes him progressively more unhappy over his relatively dependent state. He wishes to share the world of his siblings who are dating or have married and left the home. He tends to escape into a world of fantasy punctuated by violent outbursts of frustration. Communication with his parents may be totally disrupted by vocal exchanges of resentment and anger. The confused mother often handles her own ambivalence by allowing the child to punish her, thus intensifying her resentment as well as the negative self-image of the child.

Guardian

Parents are entrusted not only with the caretaking responsibility of their child but with the obligation to protect him from harm, including physical, sexual, or emotional abuse from unthinking or unscrupulous elements of the community. It is difficult for the parents to judge the extent to which they should restrict the outside activities and social contacts of their retarded child without further hindering his social development. The mildly retarded child is especially susceptible to ridicule and harassment in the school yard and by his peers in the neighborhood who may tease him or make him the butt of their jokes to enhance their own feeling of superiority. Pathetically a handicapped child may aquiesce willingly, out of a need for attention and acceptance, to playing the buffoon or becoming a dupe or scapegoat for a group of delinquent or predelinquent boys. Adolescence is a particularly difficult time for the retardate, not only because of his increased drive toward greater social interaction out of the home, but because of society's tendency to view him as sexually aggressive or potentially dangerous. It is not unusual for the retarded boy or girl at this age to begin running afoul of the law for minor misdemeanors ranging from trespassing or similar inappropriate behavior to drug use or sexually unacceptable conduct, the latter usually instigated by those who should know better but who usually manage to escape without being implicated.

Nurse

Every parent soon learns how to bandage cuts, apply nose drops, use a thermometer and attend to a number of other minor medical problems common to children. In addition to this the mother of the handicapped child must learn to handle braces and special protheses, dispense medications according to an often rigid schedule, and carry out special procedures to minimize urinary tract infections, skin ulcers, respiratory distress, and other medical problems commonly associated with brain damage and mental retardation.

Guide

Parents must guide their children through a variety of developmental crises by offering themselves as a model for identification. In this respect, parents almost compulsively tend to adopt attitudes toward training, especially as regards rejection or acceptance, permissiveness and restrictions, that closely parallel those of their own parents but which they often modify according to their own childhood experiences.* Unless they were raised in a household with a handicapped sibling, the parents of a retarded child find themselves in a strange situation where all of their attitudes, reactions, and patterns of care around toilet training, feeding, etc., must be developed *de novo*. Meanwhile the handicapped child tends to adopt the unconscious attitudes toward his handicap that his parents hold: denial, resignation, and rejection of self.

Disciplinarian

The proper balance between undercontrol and overcontrol is an area in which parents of both healthy and handicapped chil-

---

* Although the average woman is constantly engaged in a conscious effort to be different from her mother, her actual success is, in fact, often more imagined than real, especially when reacting toward various behavioral patterns in their own children. The most consistent modification is usually attained by the previously sheltered, overmothered girl who tends to go to the other extreme in adult life by becoming "liberal" and permissive with her own child.

dren have, perhaps, their greatest degree of uncertainty. No child comes into the world with the ability to tolerate frustration, postpone gratification, or to mediate his behavior so as to cope effectively with the outside world. These are the attributes of a healthy ego which are developed as a gradual process from repeated exposure to graded frustrations. Each challenge that eventuates in mastery increases the child's ability to handle further challenges. However, obstacles that are insurmountable lead only to frustration.* A child who is asked to perform beyond his capacity and then punished for failing will develop severe behavioral problems including temper tantrums, extreme avoidant withdrawal, and eventually very pathologic, rigid personality characteristics that will tend to make subsequent learning all but impossible. The other extreme is the child who, because he was sickly at birth, is overprotected and oversheltered and literally rewarded for just being alive. Such children do not learn to develop behavioral repertoires which can be used to elicit positive responses from their environment. They tend to become fearful and insecure children who shy away from any task and who may react to even moderate social or academic pressure with emotional shattering. Retarded children are especially prone to being treated at either extreme, often in alternating fashion between overexpectation and boredom. And either extreme may have the same result by either forcing or permitting the child to regress into his own self-stimulating inner world.

All discipline should be based upon a prior established positive rapport and mutual trust. However the inexperienced parent may feel the middle line becoming especially thin when dealing with adverse behavior in her retarded child, such as compulsive head-banging, masturbation, extreme negativism, and de-

---

* Parents must be advised not to try to teach their child to tolerate frustration by purposely frustrating him. This always leads to power struggles with devastating psychological consequences to both sides. (Feature your spouse refusing you a cigarette to teach you to stop smoking.) Control must come from within. An exception, of course, is the "negotiable" frustration, where the child must ask for a cookie or say "please" before receiving it. However, the danger of overdoing this teaching method must also be emphasized. There are sufficient unavoidable frustrations in the course of every normal child's day to adequately challenge his coping abilities without inventing artificial ones, except those that are amenable to easy mastery.

structive outbursts, especially when the child has severe deficits in the usual modalities of communication.

Should I Place My Child?

Every parent of a retarded child, regardless of how emotionally attached to him they may have grown or how well adjusted they had become to his needs, will almost certainly wrestle with the question of placement out of the home, if not from the beginning then at some later stage in his development. As mentioned earlier, the severely handicapped child presents a family crisis resulting in varying degrees of role disruption in all members of the family. Because, with time, changes inevitably occur in every family as well as in the individuals comprising it, the decision to institutionalize may be "time-bound" and related either to uncontrollable factors in the present situation or to changes which appear to make a previous balance untenable. The intensity of the crisis is usually less important than the pattern of stress which it imposes upon the family. These patterns may be described as follows.

Burden of Care

This involves the age and physical and emotional condition of the mother or primary caretaker, the severity of the child's handicap and his associated medical complications, the cost of medical treatment, and availability of community resources. These factors may be modified by the family size and constellation and the birth order of the retarded child. A child with Down's syndrome born to a premenopausal woman with teenage daughters in the home is less likely to present the hardships of a first-born retarded child to a young mother who has little experience in raising children and no ancillary assistance. We find that the severity of the handicaps is often a highly subjective matter, with parents who ultimately place their child tending to greatly exaggerate their child's problems in contrast to parents who keep their child at home and who tend to minimize his defects. Also, paradoxically, families that are most able financially to keep their child at home tend to have the highest rate statistically of placement in an institution.

Family Instability and Conflicts

This includes family disruption as a result of severe disciplinary problems on the part of the retardate such as temper tantrums, running away, and sexual acting-out. Tension may also arise from conflict with the neighbors, community attitudes of rejection or exclusion, and sibling jealousy and resentments. Family communication may be so strained by disagreements over the handling and care of the retardate that separation or divorce of the parents is a likely outcome. The rate of divorce between parents with a handicapped child is almost three times the national average.

Social Status and Family Expectations

A deviation is more easily accepted if it is consistent with role expectations. Thus a retarded daughter may be integrated with relative ease into a lower class family as compared to a male child with similar handicaps but in an upper middle class family. The first-born child of a young, upper mobile couple is especially likely to be institutionalized during infancy.

Religious and Philosophical Convictions of the Family

Despite the numerous reality factors enumerated above, the decision for or against placement is usually decided by subjective factors such as the religious background of the parents, and for this reason remains a highly personal matter. Professional counselors should be aware of this fact when assisting parents in the decision-making process.

SIBLINGS OF THE RETARDED

Siblings are affected, not so much by their own direct interactions with the retardate, but indirectly through the effect the retarded sibling may have on the two parents. Since children look to their parents for attention, love, guidance, and as a mirror of their own self-concept or identity, the degree to which parents are unable to fulfill their normal roles because of the burden of care of a handicapped child is the extent to which the other children become handicapped by the presence of a retarded brother or sister.

The siblings not only suffer from relative maternal deprivation because of the depletion of the mother's energies by the
care of the handicapped child and by the push toward prema-
ture independence with additional chores and responsibilities,
but also from a variety of internally and externally imposed
emotional conflicts. Their resentments toward the parents and
their anger toward the retarded brother is repressed out of guilt
at being spared, and by the fear that the handicapping condition may one day be inflicted upon them as a punishment. The
inhibition of normal, aggressive behavior is also imposed sub-
consciously by the parents. It commonly results from the children's recognition of, and unwillingness to challenge their parents' rather brittle adjustment to the ongoing stresses within the
family.

Children tend naturally to strongly adopt the attitudes and
defenses of the parents during any severe family crisis. They
will deny or believe what the parents wish and concomitantly
adopt roles which will least likely upset family cohesiveness and
stability. Many mothers manipulate the environment so that no
mention is ever made of their child's deformity or mental handicap, and the rest of the family tends to conform out of fear
and guilt to this parentally imposed "conspiracy of silence."*
The most crippling aspect of this suppression is that the parents' distorted perceptions of the sibling's attitudes and role
leaves him feeling misunderstood and inwardly dishonest.

The older children may suffer from real or imagined fears of
isolation from their peers and risk parental disapproval because
of their embarrassment and refusal to play with their retarded
brother. Siblings also frequently suffer from an increased tension between the parents. The presence of the handicapped
child in the home increases the parents' need for mutual support and hence tends to maximize preexisting communication
problems and bring to the surface long suppressed grievances

* For this reason questionnaires answered by parents concerning sibling attitudes toward a retarded brother or sister can be very misleading. In fact, the
only handicap in which parents are able to consistently verify a realistic resentment by their other children is in the case of an otherwise healthy appearing
child with congenital deafness, a defect which is less apparent and hence relatively less frightening to the other siblings.

and dissatisfactions. Differences in their perceptions of their child's handicaps as well as disagreements over the decision for placement further disrupts family solidarity. Commonly the husband will tend to become more involved in his work and in outside activities, leaving his wife with the total burden of care for all of the children. Usually the father who rejects his retarded child is subsequently unable to relate normally to any of the other children. They, in turn, become more dependent upon their mother and, in an effort to gain her attention, allow themselves to become entrapped in her orbit of special interest, the retarded sibling. They assume roles as mother's helpers, becoming parent surrogates and sometimes husband substitutes. These mothers often boast of the mature attitude of their children toward the retarded sibling, not realizing that this pseudomature facade was attained at the sacrifice of a normal childhood and very often prognosticates a severe emotional disturbance in adult life.

EMOTIONAL REACTIONS AND DEFENSE MECHANISMS OF PARENTS TOWARDS THEIR RETARDED CHILD

Parents react to the birth of a defective child with shock, disbelief, anger, disappointment, despair, and grief. This response may be intensified by the way in which they are first informed of their child's low intellectual potential. The time when the news is first received is also important. The diagnosis of mental retardation is often missed during the first few years unless it has a fairly obvious organic etiology. For one thing, there is a reluctance on the part of the physician to commit himself to this diagnosis as there still exists a pervasive feeling of pessimism among professional people regarding mental retardation. This is often related to a lack of knowledge of available treatment facilities and the physician's own feelings of helplessness and inability to offer constructive advice and support.

Sometimes what the parents are told may represent the physician's own subjective upper-middle-class attitudes toward mental retardation as an intolerable deviation within the context of our present social structure. Parents develop a variety of defenses in order to deal with this unexpected situation in which they find themselves. Many of these defenses are harmful in that they prevent them from viewing their problems realistically and only lead to further grief in the long run. Most parents are unwilling to accept the diagnosis of mental retardation, preferring to find a physical or emotional reason for their child's slow development. There also seems to be a more ominous stigma placed upon the child if he is "born that way." Sometimes parents use massive denial upon hearing the news. They might insist that they were never told that their child was retarded despite the fact that several physicians had indicated this in the past. The chief complaint is rarely, "My child is mentally retarded." Rather there is some euphemism about delayed or poor speech or not keeping up with siblings. Fathers often come in with, "This is the way I was when I was his age."

Other parents are intellectually able to accept the child as retarded but continue to react emotionally to the child as if he were not retarded and persist in maintaining unrealistic expectations of him. This condition or defense might be described as a "cognitive dissonance," where the parents, unable to emotionally accept the findings, may continually find fault with the school system, keep seeking new treatments and new medications to cure their son's condition, or pounce on the son, himself, with anger and scolding because of his "disobedience" in not performing up to standard.

When it comes to the actual handling of the child, parents react in different ways. Some may avoid direct contact with the retarded child and handle him as little as possible. Others, without deliberately rejecting the child, may detach themselves emotionally while simultaneously assuming responsibility by compulsively organizing their lives around a ritualistic schedule of care with emphasis upon cleanliness and antiseptic conditions. They tend to focus upon the child's defect rather than to perceive him as a whole person, and are often surprised later to learn that their child has many things in common with other similarly handicapped children, that someone understands and is able to redirect the aberrant behavior of their child, and that their child is capable of learning from special teaching.

Parents need recognizable feedback from their children to reinforce the continuous expenditure of time and energy toward their development. The prolongation of dependency of the retarded child, along with his need for an almost constant commitment of parental support, gradually forces the coping defenses of the parents to take on a more chronic aspect. Development of a healthy parent-child relationship is often inhibited by the establishment of a pathologic tie between mother and child, with the mother tending to orient her routine exclusively to the needs of the child. Overprotection and infantilizing attitudes toward the child gradually become an established pattern that is difficult to reverse. It also is very difficult to convince the mother that in so doing she is actually limiting and restricting her child's chances for further development.

Parents rarely can allow themselves to consciously and deliberately reject their child. However, a significant number of mothers of retarded children harbor considerable unconscious resentment and feelings of rejection toward their handicapped child. When these unconscious feelings reach a sufficiently intolerable level, the mother characteristically begins to complain about a variety of isolated tangential issues until her husband or an involved agency is manipulated into forcing her to have the child placed out of the home, a decision which she was unable to initiate independently on a conscious level.

Almost all mothers of handicapped children struggle constantly against varying degrees of guilt. Most of this guilt is based upon the fact that they are disappointed with and cannot love their child as they feel a mother should. In addition they struggle with an existential guilt that somehow they are responsible for their child's deficiencies and suffering. This guilt is handled in a variety of ways. Parents blame themselves or each other, attributing the congenital handicaps to "bad blood" or an hereditary defect on one side of the family. Needless to say, this attitude may place a permanent barrier to a healthy sexual relationship between the two parents and further impair the normal pursuit of their own emotional needs. Other parents may see the child as a punishment for past sins or as a negative aspect of their own personality. Such symbolic meanings of the retardate tend to further isolate the parents emotionally from the child and thus increase their guilt. The child may also be used negatively in problems of marital adjustment, each parent using the child as an excuse or medium to vent his own hostility toward the other.

The "martyr syndrome" is now a well-recognized pattern. The mother verbally accepts her retarded child and constantly talks about him as if welcoming the challenge to demonstrate her capacity for sacrifice and devotion. This defense can assume such proportions that in several reported cases the mother had her normal children adopted out so that she could devote herself exclusively to the needs of the handicapped child.

THERAPY WITH PARENTS AND SIBLINGS OF THE RETARDED CHILD

Any professional person sufficiently acquainted with the reality problems and emotional conflicts resulting from having and rearing a retarded child can be a potential source of therapeutic benefit to the entire family. However, many mistakes are made by inexperienced therapists whose unsolicited sympathy often serves only to intensify the parents' feelings of hopelessness and alienation. Although the parents may initially welcome the opportunity to ventilate their pent-up anxieties and grievances to a patient listener, eventually repetitious ventilation without concomitant change in their life situation tends only to increase their bitterness and sense of frustration.

But what of the parents who persist in their refusal to believe that their child is really significantly mentally retarded? This, like any other defense, should never be attacked directly. Parents will deny only that which is too painful to acknowledge consciously. We live in a mistake-oriented society where professional people are trained to focus upon pathology and then shun to treat those who irreversibly deviate too far from their concept of the ideal. It is difficult to accept a condition which society itself does not accept. It often involves a reorientation of one's own value system in terms of individual worth.

Defenses are psychological mechanisms utilized to escape supposedly unresolvable feelings resulting from situations preconceived as both intolerable and unchangeable. The therapist must be able to point out the misconception behind these preconceived ideas by offering himself as a model to gradually modify the hopeless attitude of the grieved parent toward the nature of their child's handicap. To do this the therapist must reexamine his own value system and be able to resist the temptation to believe that a low intelligence quotient makes an individual a fraction of a hypothetical ideal human being. Even severely retarded children are capable of sharing in varying degree the entire gamut of human emotion and experience. They are sensitive to their emotional environment, take pleasure from exercising their intact motor functions, enjoy music, crave attention and nurturance, express aggression, love to retrace paths of previous mastery, seek praise, and withdraw from the threat of belittlement and shame. The child must be seen as wholly "human" by the parents and still capable of participating in a satisfying human bond despite fairly severe mental retardation. Moreover the parents must realize that they are still capable of making their child happy despite his handicaps.

REFERENCES

1. Barsch, R.: *The Parent of the Handicapped Child.* Springfield, Ill., Charles C Thomas, 1968.
2. Farber, Bernard: Effects of a severely mentally retarded child on family integration. *Soc Res Child Dev (Monogr),* 24, No. 2, 1959.
3. Nichols, Peter: *Joe Egg.* New York, Grove Press, 1967.
4. Schecter, Marshall D.: The orthopedically handicapped child. *Arch Gen Psychiatr,* 4(3):247-253, 1961.

Chapter 12

MENTAL HEALTH–MENTAL RETARDATION CONSULTATION

IRWIN M. SHAPIRO

IN order to put mental health consultation as defined by Caplan,[2-4] Hume,[5-7] Parker,[8] and others[1, 10] into proper perspective, it is necessary to have some concept of community mental health in order to allow a practical approach so that priorities can be allocated to the demands on mental health and mental retardation professionals' valuable time. This makes it possible for the administrator to organize and allocate his resources. It also enables us to group health problems into manageable segments that we can both plan for and implement as funds and resources become available. As in most fields, things in community mental health seem to be divided into three parts. If I remember my Latin correctly, this began with Caesar's dividing Gaul into three parts, led to the early Christian's Trinity concept, and now we use these concepts of the Trinity for our subdivisions.

PRIMARY, SECONDARY, AND TERTIARY PREVENTION

At the level of primary prevention we would try to prevent the occurrence of a given illness. Unfortunately, in mental health, including mental retardation, we stress the number of patients being treated rather than look for the amount of illness prevented (or health maintained) in the community. The pathology model tends to keep us from focussing on primary prevention. Very few of us trained in the mental health field have spent time talking to persons at risk but without symptoms.

Secondary prevention means the treatment of acute illness, whether the first episode of acute illness or the tenth acute exacerbation of a chronic disorder. In secondary prevention we try to avoid the complications and chronicity of a disease. Unfortunately, it seems that secondary prevention is the most expensive type of prevention. As we look at American medicine, we find that we are mostly practicing secondary prevention. The health insurance concept is really sickness insurance. There is very little prevention built into health insurance plans although they are sold under this banner. It is reminiscent of the question of whether life insurance is really death insurance. Doctor Paul Lemkau once said that no disease known to mankind has ever been eradicated by treatment that is secondary prevention alone.

Tertiary prevention of illness is the prevention of the sequelae of an illness. Usually this has been thought of as a rehabilitation effort. Some of us are now thinking that perhaps this is somewhat fallacious because many of the patients presented to us in tertiary prevention have never had a successful life in the past. To talk about rehabilitating them, that is, bringing them back to their most successful functioning, is a true insult to them since their earlier functioning has been so poor.

DIRECT AND INDIRECT SERVICES

Looking at these three areas of prevention—primary, secondary, and tertiary—we can divide the modalities of treatment at each level of prevention into direct and indirect services. Let me give examples of each type.

A *direct* modality of primary prevention is the treatment of primary lues in order to avoid the tertiary stage of lues. Treating lues in the primary stages prevents the mental health breakdown associated with tertiary lues. This involves direct contact with patients. Another example is the use of a measles vaccine to prevent rubella complications in a population and thus avoid the mental retardation sequelae of that disease. The *indirect* components of primary prevention programs would be a demographic study of syphilis patients, in order to contact the primary sources and thus try to eradicate the spread of the disease. Another indirect way would be the organization of a rubella vaccine program in the community.

At the secondary level of prevention, the *direct* methods of treatment would include hospitalization, psychotherapy, psychoanalysis, and psychosomatic therapy including drugs, shock therapy, and group psychotherapy. An example of *indirect* secondary prevention would be a mental health professional's consultation work with a teacher of a disturbed adolescent in order to help the adolescent to function in school during an acute phase of illness so that he would not be designated as "retarded."

In tertiary prevention of mental illness, a *direct* service might be all the modalities available to patients of an aftercare clinic—drugs, vocational rehabilitation, occupational therapy, etc. An example of the *indirect* services available in tertiary prevention might be the community organization efforts necessary to organize a halfway house for patients being discharged from the acute treatment service or in-patient ward of a county or state hospital.

I would now like to discuss the applicability of the above scheme for understanding how mental health consultation and education fit into all three levels of prevention—primary, secondary, and tertiary. For example, mental health consultation to kindergarten teachers might help the teachers understand the separation problems of the children so that the teachers could be effective interveners in the crises that these children are going through. Their understanding of the developmental process would cut down drastically the numbers of children labelled "learning disorder." At the secondary level of prevention, the mental health consultant might be working with vocational rehabilitation counselors who are working with clients during an acute phase of an illness being treated by a mental health professional in the community. The consultant makes it possible for the counselor to continue a relationship during this acute phase of the illness and to be able to function while the counselor himself is under professional attack, as happens in the case of those who become identified as the "retarded counselors." In tertiary prevention, we might be working as consultants to a geriatric program, helping occupational therapists understand the problems of aging, in order to help their clients function to their best capacity.

MENTAL HEALTH–MENTAL RETARDATION
CONSULTATION IN NEW AGENCIES USING "CASE AIDES"

In supervising mental health consultants in training it is becoming more and more apparent that new kinds of agencies using the so-called "indigenous aide," "case aide," or what have you, are having unique types of opportunities and, therefore challenge, in the community. One of the areas that Dr. Caplan[4] speaks about as a problem to nonprofessional workers is a lack of confidence or self-esteem. As we hear examples of the kind of consultation problem being presented to consultants, it is becoming clear that lack of confidence or self-esteem is being used almost as a technique by the professionals in a given agency to keep the "aides" as a second or third-class professional rather than allowing these new workers to develop a unique role. The mental health consultant has a special opportunity with this type of agency to use the case material presented as a way of dealing with these professional rivalries and institutional conflicts.

For instance, in an agency working in a ghetto area doing a maternal and child care project with a group of high-risk* families, the workers kept presenting cases where the problem had to do with the client's inability to become independent in the community. No matter how well each individual case was handled, this theme kept recurring over and over. As in many agencies having this kind of problem, it became more and more apparent that the case material of the fight for independence represented the same fight for independence that the new professionals were having. The mental health and mental retardation consultant's role was to become an "expediter" to allow the new professionals to emerge as a potent new force in the agency.

In these new agencies, including family care homes, developmental centers, and "crisis" centers, we have the opportunity to observe mental health consultation at all three levels of preven-

---

* High-risk in this sense means families whose members are more likely to suffer breakdown with mental illness and mental retardation syndromes than would be expected in the population, for example, families who are suffering from malnutrition are more likely to have retarded children.[9]

tion. Because many of the cases have no history of "mental" breakdown we have the potential of *primary* prevention (intervention?). Some of the cases are undergoing medical treatment, which would be *secondary* prevention, and even though the medical staff will usually talk to the staff of these new agencies (and therefore the possibility for mental health consultation) very little true collaboration and mutual consultation is done. At the *tertiary* prevention level many of the nonpsychiatric agencies are the dumping ground in the community for patients who are discharged as "impossible" cases by the mental health agencies. By the use of consultation techniques these agencies and their clients can become the focus of rehabilitative efforts.

Mental health–mental retardation consultation has become the most frequently used preventive service in the United States. This modality can be used at each level of prevention. As we enter an era where conservation of resources is the battle cry, consultation can serve to tie together existing community resources and make them more useful to clients at risk in the community. Hopefully consultation can also enable new professionals in our field find their proper role.

REFERENCES

1. Berlin, I. N.: Learning mental health consultation: History and problems. *Ment Hyg,* 48:257-266, 1964.
2. Caplan, Gerald: An approach to the education of community mental health specialists. *Ment Hyg,* 43:268-280, 1959.
3. Caplan, Gerald (Ed.): *Prevention of Mental Disorders in Children.* New York, Basic Books, Inc., 1961.
4. Caplan, Gerald: *Principles of Preventive Psychiatry.* New York, Basic Books, Inc., 1964.
5. Hume, Portia Bell: Principles and practice of community psychiatry: The role and training of the specialist in community psychiatry. Bellak, Leopold (Ed.): *Handbook of Community Psychiatry and Community Mental Health.* New York, Grune and Stratton, Inc., 1964.
6. Hume, Portia Bell: Searchlight on community psychiatry. *Community Ment Health J,* 1(1):109-112, Spring, 1965.
7. Hume, Portia Bell: *The Need for Training in Community Psychiatry.* Read at the annual joint meeting of the Northern and Central California Psychiatric Societies at Tahoe City, May 20, 1961.

8. Parker, Beulah: *Mental Health In-service Training.* New York, International Universities Press, 1968.

9. President's Committee on Mental Retardation: *MR 71—Entering the Era of Human Ecology.* Washington, D.C., Department of Health, Education and Welfare, 1971.

10. Rapoport, Lydia: Consultation: An overview. In: Rapoport, Lydia (Ed.): *Consultation in Social Work Practice.* New York, Nat'l Assoc. Soc. Wrkrs., 1963, pp. 7-19.

Chapter 13

PREVENTION OF MENTAL ILLNESS IN THE MENTALLY RETARDED

Leon Cytryn and Reginald S. Lourie

CONTRARY to belief in many circles, mental retardation is no contraindication to a retarded child having normal personality development. This handicap may, however, if not handled properly, produce a greater vulnerability to emotional disturbances, which may lead in turn to any of the whole range of adjustment problems, including behavioral, neurotic, psychotic, character, and habit disorders.[7, 19, 23]

Now that there are expanding services for the retarded in the community, it becomes apparent that institutionalization is necessary chiefly for those individuals in this group who are the maladjusted or mentally ill.

This chapter attempts to identify those factors seen in practice as often providing hazards to normal personality development in the mentally retarded individual. The variety of factors which can result in retardation make it necessary to see each child as presenting his own individual combination of potential assets and liabilities. These are based on the constitutional variations any child brings to the developmental process and the way they are handled in the environment in which he grows. No effort is being made here to be comprehensive, particularly about the organically based vulnerabilities, but a few examples are selected to show the general principles involved in preventive mental health approaches. The constitutional factors selected for this discussion were singled out because they have had relatively little attention as to their implications for preventive and other clinical approaches.

The hazards to socialization, family life, and a healthy self-image have similarly been selected for presentation because these too have had relatively little discussion as part of the problems to be faced in child rearing practices with the retarded child. Finally, the interaction of these forces with the predictable stages of personality development are examined in the interests of prevention where possible distortions can occur in adjustment and functioning in the child with the handicap of retardation.

In our presentation we are concentrating mainly on the first few years of life, since any preventive work can best be accomplished during this period.[15]

CONSTITUTIONAL FACTORS*

Hypersensitivity to External and Internal Stimuli

Many mentally retarded children are unable to process and adapt to levels of sensory stimuli of more than low intensity. A rising intensity of such stimuli is perceived by the child as disturbing or even painful and can lead to behavioral disorganization.[3] Such hypersensitivity may involve one or more sensory pathways. In cases of auditory hypersensitivity, the child may perceive noises and loud voices as painful. Infants with this handicap will become upset when exposed to the sounds of a vacuum cleaner, electric shaver, radio, or television. Others cannot tolerate strong visual stimuli such as very bright and strong colors. Finally, there are infants who do not like to be touched as most infants do and show discomfort when picked up or cuddled. A failure to recognize these handicaps and to adjust the handling of the children may lead to behavioral disturbances of which the most common are hyperactivity, irritability, and avoidance.

The etiology of hyperactivity is still poorly understood and sensory hypersensitivity can be blamed for it only in some cases. Many other mentally retarded children seem to be hyperactive on a constitutional basis without having a history of such a clear-cut sensory handicap. Whatever the cause, the hyperactive mentally retarded child because of his restlessness and short at-

* See references (12) and (17).

tention span finds it particularly difficult to adapt to the already handicapped processes of learning and socialization. This behavior is disruptive to a smooth functioning of any group whether in the family, in the playground or in the classroom, and this can prevent the child's integration in such groups. The reaction of the group members to such disruption may be one of rejection, exclusion, punishment, or the disorganization of the group itself.

Irritability presents another behavioral reaction of the hypersensitive child. It may be pervasive, always present, or it may appear only in sporadic bursts at times of increased environmental or inner stimulation. This latter form of irritability is closely related to the low frustration tolerance exhibited by such children. Often, even a momentary delay in gratification, mild reprimand or blocking of undesirable behavior leads to a disorganization ranging from irritability to a violent temper tantrum. It often amounts to a total inability to tolerate even mild degrees of anxiety or uncertainty associated both with pleasant as well as unpleasant experiences. The response of the environment to such an irritable, easily frustrated child may be one of annoyance, anger, punitiveness, or exclusion. On the other hand, there may be efforts of constant appeasement, avoidance of any frustration, and, in effect, subordinating the behavior and needs of the group to every whim and mood change of the child. Both types of response tend to perpetuate and accentuate the child's low frustration threshold without affording him the opportunity to find and learn more useful ways of coping with an innate handicap.

Some children with hypersensitivity to environmental stimuli resort to a screening out behavior as if attempting to create their own artificial *Reizschutz*. Such children either avoid situations involving intense stimulation, anxiety or frustration or develop a capacity to "tune out" the environment and remain unresponsive. Whether such a defensive maneuver is adaptive depends on the degree to which the environment fails to make an impact on the child. Some capacity to avoid or screen out excessive stimulation may help the child to maintain his emotional equilibrium. However, if carried to excess, it may lead to an autistic aloofness and a creation of an invisible impenetrable wall preventing any interaction between the child and his environment.[2]

Hyposensitivity to Sensory Stimuli

A smaller proportion of mentally retarded children has an innate reduced sensitivity to incoming environment signals. In milder cases, such a stimulus barrier may be beneficial by shielding the child from stressful situations. However, a too high response threshold may lead to lack of contact with the environment and withdrawal, resulting in impairment of social responsiveness and inability to learn. It may also lead to passivity which further interferes with any social and intellectual progress.

Both above discussed groups of handicaps represent a conflict between the child's inner world and the world outside. To put it in more modern language, they represent an incongruity between input and available ways to process incoming information. It is likely that the relatively high frequency of psychotic behavior and thinking in the mentally retarded is due to such incongruity leading to a developmental arrest or regression.

Aggressive Behavior

Aggressive behavior is often seen in moderately and severely retarded children. It often takes the form of pan-aggression, directed indiscriminately toward anybody approaching the child and intruding upon his private world. In other children, the aggression is only directed toward certain people, adults or children, familiar people or strangers. The aggressive behavior may be totally unprovoked and unpredictable, and often coupled with destruction of toys, furniture, etc. Such aggressive behavior may be related to the previously related irritability and low frustration tolerance or it may be a reaction to inappropriate handling. In cases of seemingly unprovoked, unpredictable behavior a temporal lobe lesion may be present with or without accompanying epileptic seizures.

The origin of aggressive behavior is still not completely understood, but there is no doubt that pathological changes in the brain, in the form of a lesion, biochemical abnormalities or a seizure, may result in aggressive behavior both in humans and animals. On the other hand, negative environmental influences may induce aggression in a person with an intact central nervous system. The mentally retarded child is often vulnerable in both of these aspects.

The aggression of the mentally retarded child is sometimes coupled with general poor impulse control and destructive behavior. Of all undesirable behavioral traits of the mentally retarded, aggressive and destructive behavior evokes the most intensive reactions in the environment of which helplessness, anger, and a desire to eliminate the aggressive member of the family or the class are amongst the most common. No wonder that such behavior is the leading cause of institutionalization of the mentally retarded child.

The Inability to Tolerate Change

Many mentally retarded children seem unable to tolerate any change. This handicap may extend to different areas of the child's life. Sometimes, mothers of such children find it difficult to introduce new foods. A change in the environment, such as rearranging the furniture or a visit to relatives may make the child tense and upset. Any breaks or changes in the daily routine may have the same disruptive effects. The reaction of the child may range from mild irritability to a total behavioral reorganization and will depend on the extent of the handicap as well as the magnitude of the change.

EFFECTS OF MENTAL RETARDATION ON THE SOCIALIZATION PROCESS

In recent times there is a growing recognition of the importance of the early child-mother emotional ties for all future interactions with human beings.[4] The development of this crucial bond occurs in infancy, passing through an orderly sequence of such stages as the development of smiling, recognition of mother, fear of strangers, and separation anxiety. Failure to develop such a bond at that time does not preclude, but makes very difficult, the development of normal human attachments and interactions.

There is also growing recognition of the existing correlation between the general level of intelligence and the evolution of object relations and human attachments.[11] It seems that a certain minimum level of intellectual activity and comprehension is necessary to the development of meaningful human ties. The infant's recognition of his mother as an entity, separate from himself and clearly distinguishable from others, is an intellectual process which precedes or parallels its affective counterpart. This process of self-differentiation in turn depends on intact sensory and perceptual mechanisms, memory, and the ability to organize bits and pieces of information into a meaningful whole. The mentally retarded infant is highly vulnerable in all of these areas. His failure or delay in the recognition of his mother, for whatever reason, will delay (if severe, may even preclude) the development of these vital early attachments, thus slowing down and disrupting the timetable of emotional development. One such distortion is the longer duration and greater intensity of the child's dependency needs, causing a delay in developing independence and autonomy.

The phase of negativism often starts later in infancy in the retarded and lasts longer than usual, which may interfere with the process of learning and social cooperation. The prolonged period of negativism is particularly difficult for the parents to accept especially if the child's physical development is proceeding within normal limits. Inability to accept authority and to cooperate is hard to tolerate in a ten-year-old, well-developed youngster and it often marks the end-result of a bitter struggle between the parents and their retarded offspring.

INTERACTION BETWEEN THE DETERMINANTS OF BEHAVIOR

The children with Down's syndrome may possibly illustrate the interplay between genetic, social and environmental factors. As a rule, the emotional adjustment of children with Down's syndrome is better than that of children with other forms of mental retardation.[9, 10, 22] This may be because of their near normal developmental maturity in the first 6 months of life[8, 14, 21] which enables them to attain the basic stages of mother-child interaction characteristic of this crucial period and thus to acquire a solid base for all future attachments. Furthermore, these children are usually diagnosed very early, which may enable the parents to make their adjustment to the problem right at the start.

Finally, there is a possibility that children with Down's syndrome may be relatively protected from serious emotional disturbances on a genetic basis. In this connection, the recently described abnormalities of the biogenic amines in Down's syndrome are of great interest, but require further clarification.[21]

Disruptive Family Relationships

Rejection is probably the most damaging but most common reaction of family members to the mentally retarded individual. A mentally retarded family member threatens the image of family adequacy, undermines the parents' self-esteem and demands a central position in the family's activities and orientation.[1] Parents with low self-esteem are particularly prone to perceive the mentally retarded child as a threat to their security. If the marriage is stable and based on mutual trust and respect, the impact of a defective child will be lessened and his chances of acceptance increased.

Overprotection on the part of the parent of his mentally retarded child is frequently regarded as a reaction formation to the feeling of rejection, unacceptable to the parent's moral code. In fact, rejection and overprotection are often seen as two sides of the same coin. Clinical experience makes one doubt the universality of such a theoretical concept. There are certainly parents who overprotect their mentally retarded child not because of inner hostility (or defense against it) but because of anxiety or exaggerated feeling of compassion. Other parents may want to overcompensate for the rejection of the child by their spouse. Finally, there are lonely people with little sense of accomplishment or satisfaction who find in the care of their mentally retarded child a sense of purpose which was previously missing from their lives. Such people view the care of their child not as a parental task but rather as an all-encompassing mission, and their zeal may lead to distortions.

The recent interest in the family process and family therapy often focuses on the concept of the family scapegoat. Where there is tension, mistrust, resentment, and lack of communication, it is often the different and burdensome family member who is singled out to drain off the family's tension and the mentally retarded child is particularly vulnerable to become the prime target. Scapegoating permits the other family members not to face their own difficulties and fosters the belief that all their problems are caused by the troublemaker. For a mentally retarded child, the position of a family scapegoat may be devastating by inducing feelings of guilt, inadequacy, and worthlessness.

Low Self-Esteem

The growing mentally retarded child becomes progressively aware of being different from other normal people. Such an awareness may result from an evaluation and comparison of his performance to that of other members of his family or social group. On the other hand, it may be a reflection of the negative evaluation of the mentally retarded child by people in his environment. The brighter, mildly retarded individual is more prone to view himself as inadequate, damaged or bad, while the more retarded individual lacks the capacity for introspection and objective evaluation of his performance. The feeling of inadequacy and low self-esteem may lead to overt depression with attendant psychomotor retardation and social withdrawal. Sometimes the depression may be masked and will be expressed in depressive equivalents such as delinquent antisocial behavior, disruptive classroom behavior, hyperactivity, or physical symptoms. The mentally retarded adolescent is particularly vulnerable to feelings of inadequacy and poor self-image. His developing intellect permits more accurate self-evaluation and his progressive loneliness, as his neighborhood play companions and siblings surpass him one by one, makes denial of his inferiority difficult or impossible.

PREVENTION OF MENTAL ILLNESS

As in normal children, the foundations of personality development in mentally retarded children are laid in the first five years of life. It is particularly important to insure proper resolution of the dependency needs since if not properly solved, the child can remain preoccupied with having these needs met throughout life. In the authors' opinion, this phase of development is best handled in the child's home, and removal from home at an early age is usually counterindicated, except under unusual circumstances such as severe parental neglect or abuse or other serious family pathology. Even in such cases, efforts should be made to place the child in foster care rather than in an institution.

Early Recognition of Mental Retardation

Mental retardation is unrecognized in many children until their second or third year of life. The children may look normal at birth and, barring severe prenatal, paranatal, or postnatal complications, their retardation may not even be suspected. Thus the parents are prepared for normal development, behavior, and reaction to the environment. These expectations, however, are soon thwarted and frustrated. To begin with, the children often fail to smile and to respond to the overtures of their parents. They may be irritable, restless, and present sleeping and feeding difficulties. Finally, as the children grow, delays in their motor and speech development are becoming progressively more apparent. Many parents are bewildered by these unexpected phenomena and after a while begin to seek professional advice. Their search for clarification is frequently frustrated by well-meaning physicians who often reassure them that the child is a "late bloomer" and "will outgrow it." These false reassurances help to convince the parents that the child is "stubborn" and contrary. They intensify their efforts but the child does not reward them, and a conflict begins which often distorts the parent-child relationship for years to come. Soon the parents begin to shop from physician to physician to search for an answer. Finally, usually in the second or third year of the child's life, someone diagnoses mental retardation which by then can no longer be denied. The parents' reactions very often encompass shock as well as relief brought by certainty, however painful. The parents vividly describe their feelings of frustration, anger, guilt, and dashed hopes during the time preceding the definitive diagnosis.

In contrast, an early diagnosis forces the parents to come to grips with the problem in a realistic manner, and to gear their expectations to the child's true potential. This in turn fosters adjustment and reduces frustration and tension.

A parallel phenomenon exists in other chronic handicapping conditions. For instance, children with congenital amputation have much fewer emotional disturbances than those with cystic fibrosis. The parents of the latter group often experience years of uncertainty and anguish preceding an ultimate diagnosis that finally confirms their growing suspicion that "something is wrong."[5]

Thus, we believe that an early diagnosis of mental retardation could improve the chances for a harmonious parent-child relationship. This calls for a greater familiarity on the part of pediatricians and family physicians with normal and abnormal signs of the physical and social child development. Developmental evaluations routinely included in a periodic health check-up would sharpen the physician's diagnostic acumen and heighten his index of suspicion.

Of course, there are many situations where mental retardation cannot be ruled out or diagnosed with certainty, except after a reasonably long follow-up. These are often the most difficult cases to handle and require a combination of professional honesty and caution from the physician. He should share with the parents his concerns and suspicions without alarming them unduly. His emotional support of the parents is particularly crucial in such cases of prolonged uncertainty.

Physician's Guidance in Handling the Child's Vulnerabilities

Having arrived at a proper diagnosis, the physician is in a good position to guide the parents through the early life of the child with a minimum of distortion. If the child exhibits hypersensitivity to external stimuli, the parents will be advised to lower the intensity of such stimuli in the child's environment, and strive toward a calm atmosphere and a low-key sensory stimulation. On the other hand, parents of a child with hyposensitivity will be advised to intensify sensory stimulation in order to reach the child. The child's inability to handle frustration and anxiety will be explained as an innate handicap rather than willful misbehavior and parents should be directed toward efforts to minimize anxiety-producing situations as much as possible.

The physicians' familiarity with the natural history of some innate handicaps such as hypersensitivity to sensory stimuli helps him to reassure the parents that in most instances this will diminish or disappear altogether with advancing age. Some modern findings coming from the field of endocrinology may possibly shed light on this phenomenon. Certain glandular insufficiencies such as that of the adrenal cortex and parathyroid are often associated with a curious combination of hypersensitivity to various sensory stimuli coupled with an inability to interpret the incoming information in a meaningful way. For instance, some patients with adrenocortical insufficiency develop hypersensitivity to sound but are unable to understand speech. Restitution of hormonal balance by appropriate treatment results in a disappearance of the sensory handicap.[13]

Another interesting phenomenon is the irritability and hyperactivity of babies whose mothers were treated with female sex hormones during pregnancy. The present research interest in the origins and prevention of violence will hopefully contribute to our better understanding and management of the aggressive mentally retarded individual.

Preparation of a mother for a delay in the child's responses to her social overtures will reduce her disappointment, guilt, and pain and ensure her continuous involvement with the child, thus preventing her emotional withdrawal so often seen in parents of retarded children. The parents have to be impressed with the importance of social stimulation which uses any of the available avenues of reaching the child, such as talking, smiling, holding, cuddling, bouncing, carrying, and many others. Of equal importance is the avoidance of such avenues which tend to make the child uncomfortable. If this is not done, the child will associate closeness to human beings with discomfort and pain and will tend to withdraw from any intensive interaction.

Our primary emphasis must be on helping the child to emerge

from the primitive state of primary autism and to establish a bond of closeness between mother and child. There are, however, further hazards which can be avoided by appropriate preparation of the family. One such hazard is the failure to recognize the need of a mentally retarded toddler to be close to his mother, to shadow her, follow her around the house and even cling to her physically. Margaret Mahler described this need as naturally occurring in normal children at the age of 18 to 24 months and called it "rapprochement."[16] Because of the previously mentioned distorted timetable of personality development, the mentally retarded may not reach this stage until the age of 3, 4 or even 5, often after having achieved considerable autonomy. The frantic mother who put so much effort in teaching the child to be independent, often views such regressive clinging with alarm and fears a total breakdown of already established patterns. She may fail to respond to the child's approaches and indeed views with annoyance and discouragement his awkward efforts to be close to her. A timely prediction of such regressive behavior and its desirability for normal personality development may prevent maternal frustration and a mother-child struggle which would lead to a fixation of regressive, clinging behavior on the part of the child or turning away and withdrawal from social interaction, sometimes coupled with a chronic depressive mood.

Another hazard already mentioned resulting from the distorted timetable of personality development is the delayed onset and prolonged duration of the phase of negativism in the mentally retarded individual. This phase, if mishandled, may give rise to strong parent-child conflicts even in case of normal development. However, the hazards of devastating, protracted battles between parent and child are far greater in the mentally retarded. Parents have to be guided to avoid "head-on collisions" and be selective in placing emphasis on disciplinary matters. They need help to sail the sometimes narrow isthmus between the Scylla of overpunitiveness and the Charybdis of overindulgence and lack of control.

What is often of crucial importance is the parent's realization that it is risky to leave things to chance in the hope that the mentally retarded individual will amuse himself and keep busy. Experience shows that even the most irritable and difficult youngsters will do much better if their day is planned. Furthermore, they do better in a one-to-one relationship. Since this is next to impossible for one person to provide, one would stress the need for having the burden shared on a regular basis by family members and baby-sitters.

Enhancing the Self-Image of the Mentally Retarded Child

Acceptance by his parents despite his uniqueness is the best assurance of an adequate self-image of the mentally retarded individual. An opportunity for learning and developing social, academic, vocational, and motor skills in a good school setting is also essential. As the child grows older, a steady job, however simple, and regularly scheduled tasks contribute to a feeling of self-dignity, belonging, and identity. They also foster good social habits and a sense of responsibility.

The social isolation of the mentally retarded adolescent and young adult is best prevented by a provision of appropriate social outlets such as recreational centers with regularly scheduled, supervised activities. Contemporary thinking considers early confinement of the mentally retarded individual in an institution as often detrimental to social, emotional, and intellectual development. However, as institutions change and improve they may be very useful in certain situations. One of these is the mentally retarded child in a very disturbed family with little capacity for change. Such youngsters may be happier and better adjusted away from their troubled home. Another situation may involve a retarded adolescent living in a community without adequate social and recreational opportunities. In such a case, the alternative to institutional placement may be total social isolation, for which even a loving home atmosphere may not always compensate.

In addition, other facilities may serve the needs of mildly retarded individuals who cannot be cared for at home, yet do not require a full-time residential center. The halfway houses may be ideally suited for adolescent and adult mildly retarded individuals who require a minimum of supervision and who can work in the community or in sheltered workshops.

Finally, a word should be said about the need to prevent the detrimental often dehumanizing effects of the old fashioned state institutions which actually fostered regressive and even psychotic behavior. Modern institutional concepts stress education and training rather than custodial care. A homelike setting instead of sterile barracks and an adequate staff are absolutely essential in fostering good social behavior and self-dignity of the patients. This, plus close contact with the family and the community at large, will maximize mental health and prevent institutions from becoming dumping grounds for social rejects, instead of places of rehabilitation.

Family Counseling

Most parents need only an understanding and supportive physician who does not consider his role as completed as soon as he announces the diagnosis, but who remains involved, helping the parents to share the burden and guiding them through the difficult phases of bringing up a retarded child.[18] Such a physician will use tact, while dealing with the feelings of the parents, while at the same time being frank and honest. Allowances have to be made for the parents' grief, shattered hopes, shame and guilt which may be present at one time or another and have to be dealt with, lest they intrude on the parent-child relationship, or on other relationships within the family. The parents' helplessness is best handled by giving them specific things to do and by stressing their crucial role in helping the child to develop as normal a personality as possible.

The approach to parents has to be flexible and pragmatic. Judiciously used support, reassurance, guidance, and practical advice as to the management of the child are often indicated. Homemaking services, temporary placement of the child in institutions, and similar arrangements increase the parents' effectiveness by giving them periodic relief. This in turn enhances the family's acceptance of its mentally retarded individual. Preventive group therapy which permits the sharing of burdens and getting reassurance from similarly afflicted parents is especially effective with parents of retarded children. Parents should also be encouraged to participate in social action on behalf of the retarded. Such social action is mainly responsible for the recent public interest and progress in the field of mental retardation. In addition, it provides the parents with an outlet for useful activity which decreases their frustration and despair.

Effective parent counseling by the physician requires his thorough knowledge of the appropriate community agencies and resources in his area, such as educational facilities, institutions, vocational rehabilitation, public school classes for the retarded and sheltered workshops.

The foregoing recommendations regarding prevention of mental illness in the mentally retarded, call for an involvement and central role of the family physician and pediatrician. Unfortunately, even today, the subject of mental retardation receives only short attention in many medical schools and residency programs. To remedy this situation requires making the modern knowledge about various aspects of retardation an integral part of the medical curriculum.[6] The problem is too vast to be left in the hands of a few "super-specialists." Other disciplines like psychology, nursing, and social work share in the guilt of neglect of this vital area. Without vigorous professional support, any attempt to prevent mental illness in the mentally retarded is not very likely to succeed.

REFERENCES

1. Begab, M. J.: *The Mentally Retarded Child: A Guide to Services of Social Agencies.* Washington, D.C., U.S. Department of Health, Education and Welfare, Children's Bureau, 1963.
2. Bender, L.: Autism in children with mental deficiency. *Arch Neurol Psychiatr,* 63:81, 1959.
3. Bergman, P. and Escalona, S. K.: Unusual sensitivities in very young children. *Psychoanal Study Child,* 3(4):333-352, New York, International Universities Press, 1969.
4. Caldwell, B. M.: The usefulness of the critical period hypothesis in the study of filiative behavior. *Merrill-Palmer Quart,* 8:229-242, 1962.
5. Cytryn, L.: Factors in psychosocial adjustment of children with chronic illness. *Clin Proc Child Hosp (DC),* 27:7, 200-210, 1971.
6. Cytryn, L.: The training of pediatricians and psychiatrists in mental retardation. In Menolascino, F. J. (Ed.): *Psychiatric Approaches to Mental Retardation.* New York, Basic Books, Inc., 1970.
7. Cytryn, L. and Lourie, R. S.: Mental retardation. In Friedman, A. M.

and Kaplan, H. J. (Eds.): *Comprehensive Textbook of Child Psychiatry.* Baltimore, Md., Williams and Wilkins, 1967.

8. Dameron, L. E.: Development of intelligence of infants with mongolism. *Child Dev,* 34:733, 1963.

9. Domino, G., *et al.:* Personality traits of institutionalized mongoloid girls. *Am J Ment Defic,* 68:498, 1969.

10. Ellis, A. and Beechley, R. M.: A comparison of matched groups of mongoloid and non-mongoloid feebleminded children. *Am J Ment Defic,* 54:464, 1950.

11. Guin-Decarie, T.: *Intelligence and Affectivity in Early Childhood.* New York, International Universities Press, 1965.

12. Heider, D. M.: Vulnerability in infants and young children: A pilot study. *Gene Psychol Monogr,* 73:1-216, 1966.

13. Henkin, R. I.: The Neuroendocrine Control of Perception. In Hamburg, D. (Ed.): *Perception and Its Disorders.* Baltimore, Md., Williams and Wilkins, 1970.

14. Koch, R., *et al.:* Gesell development scales in mongolism. *J Pediatr,* 62:93, 1963.

15. Lourie, R. S.: The first 3 years of life. *Am J Psychiatr,* 127:11, 1971.

16. Mahler, M.: Notes on the Development of Basic Mood, the Depressive Affect. In Lowenstein, R. M., Newman, L. M., Shurr, M., and Solnit, A. J. (Eds.): *Psychoanalysis: A General Psychology.* New York, International Universities Press, 1966.

17. Murphy, L. B.: Problems in Assessment of Infants and Young Children. In Dittmann, L., Lourie, R. S., and Chandler, C. A. (Eds.): *New Perspectives in Early Child Care.* New York, Atherton Press, 1969.

18. Paine, R. S. and Cytryn, L.: Counselling parents of mentally retarded children. *Clin Proc Child Hosp* (D.C.), 21:106, 1965.

19. Philips, I.: Psychopathology and mental retardation. *Am J Psychiatr,* 124:29, 1967.

20. Rosner, F., *et al.:* Biochemical differentiation of trisomic Down's Syndrome (mongolism) from that due to translocation. *New Eng J Med,* 273:1356, 1965.

21. Share, T., *et al.:* Longitudinal development of infants and young children with Down's Syndrome. *Am J Ment Defic,* 68:685, 1964.

22. Silverstein, A. B.: An empirical test of the mongoloid stereotype. *Am J Ment Defic,* 68:493, 1969.

23. Webster, T. G.: Unique Aspects of Emotional Development in Mentally Retarded Children. In Menolascino, F. J. (Ed.): *Psychiatric Approaches to Mental Retardation.* New York, Basic Books, Inc., 1970.

Chapter 14

WHAT IS A SUCCESSFUL SEXUAL ADJUSTMENT FOR THE MENTALLY RETARDED?

Virginia Y. Blacklidge

THE sexual life of a retarded person depends on where he lives and who is in control. A meaningful sexual relationship is the most intimate relationship possible between two persons and a successful sexual adjustment maximizes the amount of intimacy possible or comfortable between two persons. The mentally retarded have the same desire and need as normal people for intimate relationships with others, but this is not the same as saying they have the same sexual needs as others.

Intimacy, as referred to here, was defined by Eric Berne[4] as the direct, honest expression of meaningful emotions between two people, without any tricks (ulterior motives, reservations, or games). Most infants, retarded and otherwise, seem to be naturally loving and able to enjoy intimacy until experience causes them to relate differently, that is, until their desires conflict with those around them, who, in turn, do not react so lovingly. Since the retarded child takes longer to grow up and needs more physical care in his younger years, his needs are likely to conflict more with those around him.

Most retarded children become convinced that they are inferior long before they reach adult life. Among the mildly retarded, Morgenstern[13] showed that the higher the functioning intelligence, the more critical the self-appraisal.

Sustained intimacy occurs between two people (retarded or not) who, viewing themselves as lovable, are essentially equals or have something equally valuable to offer the relationship. If one person feels inferior, unimportant or not valuable, he will

194

eventually try to put the other into an inferior position so that he feels better by comparison. Sustained love requires that the lover love himself first.

THE PROFOUNDLY RETARDED

For many profoundly retarded the opposite of intimacy—withdrawal—is their predominant relationship, not because of the degree of retardation but rather because of the way they have been treated by others (mainly ignored). If not withdrawal, many profoundly retarded take refuge in some sort of ritualistic banging and grunting. This relieves boredom and makes time seem to go faster. This is acquired behavior. Much of the banging and grunting disappears when the profoundly retarded are placed in good homes or convalescent hospitals where the level of personal, loving care is superior to that in the usual state hospital or many natural homes.

> In Alameda County, California, there is a convalescent hospital which was built to take care of nonambulatory retarded as well as sick adults and geriatric patients. When six profoundly retarded children with a mental age under one year were placed there from a state hospital in 1969, three made incessant, irritating, whining noises. The nursing staff enjoyed taking care of these obviously helpless children (even more than caring for sick adults) and gave them much more attention than they had previously been receiving. Within four months, the obnoxious whines had stopped.*

For the profoundly retarded, the most intimate relationship will of necessity be with the mother or caretaker and this is not usually thought of as a sexual relationship. However, this can be a very meaningful experience to a lonely mother or caretaker and it may take the place of more usual sexual experiences for her. The intensity of this relationship from the retardate's point of view is unknown, but it is relatively easily transferred to other caretakers.

THE MODERATELY AND SEVERELY RETARDED

For the moderately and severely retarded, who are also dependent on a mother or caretaker for some of their needs, their

---

* Contractures of hips, knees, elbows, and wrists were also lessened and feeding became easier.

closest relationship is likely to be with the parent or caretaker unless this person is rejecting or hostile. In this case, the retardate may seek a close relationship among others outside the home. If this happens, the object of intimacy is likely to change from time to time because the rejected retarded person's feeling of unworthiness makes it difficult for him to have long-time friends. A duty-bound family which takes care of a retarded member even when relationships are not harmonious may unknowingly interfere with the retarded person's adjustment at out-of-home activities.

It is fortunate that the severely retarded can adjust with relative ease to changing objects of intimacy since many of them are moved from one home or institution to another several times during a lifetime and yet many seem to make the adjustment without profound mental illness and many gain greater mental health. It is often said that it is harder for the former parent or guardian to adjust to the loss of a loved retarded person than it is for the retardate himself.

In general, the more retarded a person is, the less he will seek sexual relationships with others. Some people believe this is because the retarded are protected from sexual relationships with others. However, even where the opportunity exists for intermingling with the opposite sex, the majority of those who take advantage of the opportunity for sexual relationships are higher in ability than those who do not.

Sexual intercourse is unlikely to be initiated by the severely retarded in a nonsexually stimulating environment. However, the severely retarded, like the rest of us, can be sexually aroused by provocative circumstances, and once aroused they are likely to have less control over their emotions than more capable persons. People with a mental age four to eight years are not noted for their emotional control. Fun for the moment is not weighed against future problems.

Exposure

The severely retarded can be sexually provocative without knowing it if untrained or unsupervised—like the retarded man who dressed and undressed in front of a large glass window when the neighbor's teen-age children were near the other side. He had simply not been trained to dress and undress in private. Once the retarded person learns that exposure of private parts draws attention, he may continue, just to get attention. Negative attention is better than none at all.

Exposure of private parts may occur when a child is "dared" by his peers and he feels impelled to follow through in order to win their respect.

> Greg was transferred from one educable mentally retarded (EMR) class to another in a different elementary school at age twelve. Three months later he was recognized as the least capable child in the class and he was learning so slowly that gains were almost imperceptible. Two of his classmates "dared" him to pull his pants down and he did. Despite temporary suspension for this, he again exposed himself on the playground twice a week later.
>
> His middle class parents were shocked at his behavior and equally upset by his lack of progress in the classroom. These episodes brought him to the school psychologist's attention. He was retested and found to have an IQ in the 40's. He was soon transferred to a trainable retarded (TMR) class more suited to his level of functioning.

Fertility

The fertility of the severely retarded is often said to be less than that of normal persons. Follow-up studies on the number of children produced by severely retarded parents report that only 3 per cent of the moderately and severely retarded have children. The severely retarded are seldom married and usually live in a sheltered environment because they cannot take care of all their own personal needs. The reduced fertility appears to be more a factor of reduced incidence of sexual intercourse rather than a biologic inability to reproduce. Accurate data have never been published on how frequently the moderately and severely retarded engage in sexual intercourse.

Mongoloid women (the majority of whom are moderately or severely retarded) are known to be capable of reproducing and 50 per cent of their offspring are Mongoloid. So far there are no published reports of offspring of Mongoloid men. When men are unmarried their offspring are hard to identify. In one study the fertility of moderately and mildly retarded men discharged from a state school was almost half that of retarded women even though one-sixth as many men had been sterilized.[20]

Masturbation

While interpersonal sexual relationships are unlikely to be initiated by the severely retarded, the same is not true for erotic self-stimulation. Most severely retarded persons outside of institutions spend considerable time alone, and it does not take much intellect to discover that certain parts of the body give pleasurable feelings when manipulated. Even when not alone, the bored retardate will explore his private parts for some way to relieve the boredom or for lack of meaningful (to him) activity. This is simply taking advantage of one's natural resources. Some masturbation in private is healthy and to be expected.

If masturbation occurs by the hour, there is a need for additional constructive ways to occupy the time.

> Gary was a thirteen-year-old severely retarded boy housed in a temporary county court facility where he "didn't fit into the group." He was placed in "isolation" with only a mattress in the room and spent nearly all his waking hours masturbating, rocking, and enjoying other kinds of self-stimulation. When I visited, he took my hand to rub his back. After he was placed in a foster home, he learned to keep his pants on and was only rarely observed to masturbate.

Masturbation occurs secondarily when there is nothing more exciting to do. The amount of masturbation present in a classroom, workshop, home, or institution is an index of how much the intellectual and/or emotional needs of the retarded are being met. A teacher or caretaker who is successful in keeping her charge's attention and interest has no significant problem with masturbation. To eliminate masturbation in public, a more worthwhile activity must be found which is as enjoyable or more enjoyable. This is a real challenge to persons caring for the retarded.

Homosexuality

Sporadic invitations to participate in male homosexual experiences are available for the retarded and nonretarded in most public rest rooms and high school locker rooms. The retarded boy is likely to be more gullible, more easily coerced, bribed, or blackmailed into participating. If living in all-male or all-female quarters (such as a state institution) the provocation to homosexual behavior is vastly increased. The lack of close personal relationships, boredom, and often a shortage of supervisory personnel make homosexual activity more common in institutions, whether the institutions are for the retarded, the delinquent, private boarding school pupils, or the military.

Retarded teen-age boys, even more than normal teen-age boys, need to be prepared for a homosexual proposition. This suggestion comes as a shock to some mothers who feel unprepared to give the necessary education and then try to provide additional protection for their sons. Fathers are generally less accepting of homosexual behavior than mothers. Some urge their sons into heterosexual relationships after known incidents of homosexual relations.

Most homosexual relationships are sporadic and emotionally superficial. They are a "quickie" arrangement without future commitment. The lonely retarded boy may wish a longer relationship if the initial encounter is pleasurable and he may then be taken advantage of emotionally and/or financially. The severely and moderately retarded are especially vulnerable to homosexuality because they are more frequently lonely and easily persuaded, and more often placed in institutions. As boys, they are also likely to have been closer to their mothers than their fathers and more often overprotected by their mothers.

ENCOURAGING APPROPRIATE SEXUAL BEHAVIOR

If the severely retarded are to understand what is appropriate sexual behavior they need to see, hear, and feel it. They have difficulty learning a set of rules which is different from what is practiced around them. For maximum responsible sexual behavior, they will need to exercise responsibilities in other areas too. Every year they can be a little more responsible and independent than the year before, if this is expected by those with whom they live. Often overzealous parents or caretakers do more for the retarded than is necessary. They do this because the retarded are slow and they can do it faster, or because it requires too much patience to show the retarded how. They do not see the value to the retarded person of doing something himself. The severely retarded person who is as independent as possible will have a better opinion about himself and relate better to others.

Living Arrangements

It is fortunate for the emotional and intellectual development of the retarded that there has been a trend toward keeping young retarded children and school-aged retarded children at home. The older the child gets, the more different he is from others the same age. When public school is no longer available, at age 18 to 21 years, it is worth considering whether the moderately and severely retarded adult will benefit more from remaining at home than from living elsewhere. At home he is likely to be more protected. Experience with many retarded adults who have lived both in their own homes as well as boarding homes or foster homes has impressed me with the increased happiness most retarded adults gain when they get to live away from home.

This increased happiness comes not only from feeling grown up when they can live away from home but also because living away from home usually means living with their retarded peers with whom they feel comfortable. When they are not the only handicapped person in the home, there is less likelihood that they will feel they are interfering with the happiness of others.

Residences for the adult retarded used to be very scarce. Now they are more common. Residences which include both children and adults allow a broader experience than those which include only children or adults.

Some single or married retarded women would likely have less desire for children of their own if they could help "mother" other children. In instances where offspring are not possible or not planned, caring for other children could provide a healthy additional dimension for retarded adults. A cluster of homes, some for handicapped children and some for handicapped adults, or just good neighbors, could give this breadth of experience.

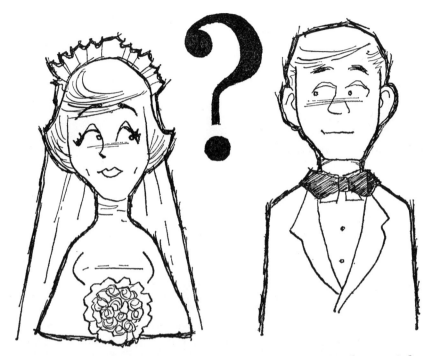

Figure 4. Marriage for the mentally retarded. From *Sexual Behavior of the Mentally Retarded*, by Virginia Blacklidge. Courtesy of the author.

THE MILDLY RETARDED

The sexual interests and fertility of the mildly retarded (those with a mental age of 7 to 11 years as adults) approximate those of the intellectually normal.

For the mildly retarded a sustained relationship with someone other than the mother or caretaker is more possible not only because of fewer physical needs that must be satisfied by someone else, but also because the seven-to-eleven-year-old mind seeks relationships outside the home. This is the age of secret groups and select clubs that provide status among peers.

Most mildly retarded persons become self-supporting. In good economic times about 75 per cent are successful in getting and keeping jobs. The self-supporting retarded logically think in terms of marriage like other self-supporting adults in our society where the norm for healthy adults is marriage. It is often easier, however, to keep a job than it is to keep a wife or husband, because of the difference in the nature of the relationship.

MARRIAGE AND OTHER HETEROSEXUAL RELATIONSHIPS

Sometimes marriage is considered because of the status this will give without understanding the degree of intimacy needed to keep such a relationship alive.

> Pat, a nineteen-year-old black girl on leave from a state hospital for the retarded, lived with her elderly grandmother who had reared her. She married a 35-year-old uneducated, unskilled laborer with no savings. He moved into grandma's two-bedroom apartment with Pat, who then refused to sleep with him or otherwise allow him to relate to her sexually.

An intimate relationship is the most demanding of all relationships and many adults, retarded or not, fail either to achieve such a relationship or to maintain it. (The current divorce rate in California is about 50 per cent.) What is difficult for the normal person is doubly difficult for the retarded person who has fewer resources at his command.

Therefore, the ideal marriage relationship is not possible for many retarded persons and this is likely to be difficult for them to understand. When the retarded also have some physical handicap (such as cerebral palsy, epilepsy, blindness, or deafness), it is easier to help them understand that a good marriage is not possible. This is much more difficult to explain to an emotionally disturbed, retarded person.*

The mildly retarded, like the severely retarded, learn more easily by experience than by being told how. Unfortunately, it is difficult to teach marriage relationships by experience. Lucky are those few whose own parents have had an ideal marriage which can be used as a model. Those retarded who can marry and rear one or two children successfully are those who are happy before marriage, have "good" parent marriages, know their

---

* The retarded, like other brain injured persons, have about twice the incidence of serious emotional disturbance as normal people, according to Rutter *et al.*[18]

abilities and limitations, know when and how to ask for advice, and have a good income. Such persons would have reasonably good control over their emotions and near-maximum development of innate ability.

Sheltered living arrangements (hostels or boarding homes) need to be established for some married retarded couples unable to live independently. Such quarters could provide supervision, meals, recreation, medication, money management, and counseling when needed. Supervision might include making sure working persons got up on time, and that personal hygiene was up to standard. Without such an arrangement the mildly retarded with an additional handicap are likely to have a stormy life and many hurts.

Casual or secret sexual relationships outside of marriage have special difficulties for the retarded. The retarded have more difficulty keeping secrets, and are more easily taken advantage of by pimps and madames in houses of prostitution.

In a state hospital with unlocked wards and large grounds, sexual relationships may occur with or without the knowledge of the ward staff. Some hospital employees feel the retarded deserve a little something extra to make life more enjoyable and do not report all "incidents." When a retarded person accustomed to sexual experiences is placed back into the community, where most foster parents and boarding home operators do not condone sexual relationships, he is likely to run into difficulty which may necessitate his return to a state hospital.

At present, disproportionally large numbers of retarded persons are living in poor housing and on welfare or in subwelfare conditions. This means that a relatively large proportion of the mildly retarded practice the sexual life style of the poor. Sexual productivity may be the primary productivity outlet for these poor and there is a sense of fullfilment in using one's body for this type of production. Then too, there is always the hope that the new baby's life will be better than that of the parents, and the parents can enjoy that vicariously.

THE MILDLY RETARDED PARENT

In order to decide whether or not to have children, the retarded need to assess their ability to care for children satisfactorily and their risk of giving birth to a handicapped child. Among the mildly retarded, success in child rearing depends less on their degree of retardation than on their emotional adjustment and the number of children they have. In other words the amount of intelligence is less important than how well the intelligence is used. The "IQ" by itself is not an accurate predictor of a person's future achievements. An emotionally well-adjusted person of IQ 50 may be more productive and successful than an emotionally disturbed person of IQ 70. An emotionally well-adjusted retarded person would not want to produce more children than he could care for emotionally and financially.

The risk of producing additional handicapped children is not likely to be considered at all unless there is parental or professional guidance. Generally a retarded person does not think it unfortunate to produce a retarded child unless that child turns out to be more handicapped than the parent.

If a person is retarded because of an illness or accident, his children probably will be born with normal mentality if his mate is normal or retarded for the same reason. It does not matter whether the illness or accident occurs before birth, after birth, or in childhood. However, if the retardation is hereditary, the offspring will have an increased likelihood of being retarded from the moment of birth.

Most studies of the causes of retardation conclude that in the vast majority of cases the cause is unknown or uncertain. There are families with a disproportionately large number of mentally retarded members, but many of these persons have had inadequate or no prenatal care, poor diet, untreated neonatal and childhood illness, unrecognized partial deafness, childhood accidents, poisonings, or lack of love and early stimulation. If medical and paramedical care were more readily available to the poor and undereducated, the incidence of retardation would probably drop in many families.

Because the author works in a public clinic for the retarded in need of help, her personal experience has been mostly with unsuccessful retarded parents. Among the 75 per cent of mildly retarded who are employed (and then lose their "retarded" label), the child rearing success probably approaches that of normal employed people.

Eugene was a severely retarded hyperactive boy who was provocative and noisy at school. When his mildly retarded mother was approached about getting help for him she couldn't understand why the school had problems with him when she didn't. She thought the school was inferior since it was a school for the retarded. She said Eugene was as smart as she was.

She had been hospitalized 3 years previously for alcoholism and found at that time to have an IQ of 60. She had had two children out of wedlock as a teenager and these were being raised by her mother in another state. Her husband of fourteen years was steadily employed and able to provide for their four children. They were preparing to move into a home they were buying.

Eugene was placed on a mild stimulant with instructions that it be taken only at school to insure its regular intake. His behavior at school improved dramatically.

Many retarded women get pregnant accidentally, and some girls pretend they are not pregnant in hopes that this will cause the pregnancy to go away. People who do not believe they are pregnant do not seek abortions, just as girls who do not believe they will ever have sexual relations do not use birth control.

Some retarded women want children because of imagined benefits accruing to the status of parenthood.

Maria, a nineteen-year-old mildly retarded woman, home after five years in a state hospital, had difficulty getting along with her mother who disapproved of her boyfriends. She had a daughter by a man who was not interested in marrying her, though she kept hoping he would change his mind. She and her daughter lived on welfare funds in various housing projects. From age three to five years the daughter attended a nursery school while her mother got job training. This training never materialized into a job. When the daughter began public school, attendance was irregular because her mother overslept. She enjoyed the late movies on television and entertained her boyfriends far into the morning. The child often told people at school that she didn't have food to eat at home and was scared by her mother's boyfriends. At age seven years the court took custody of the daughter and awarded her to the maternal grandmother. In the first nine months after the daughter was taken away from her, Maria attempted suicide three times with an overdose of her anticonvulsant medication.

Maria used her daughter as an excuse to live independently. She said many times how glad she was that she had a daughter and that she would like to have more children. She had no understanding that her child-rearing techniques needed to be improved.

Some married or single retarded parents do such a poor job raising children that the courts have to take custody of the children to place them out of the home. This does not improve the mental health of the retarded parent. If a retarded couple has difficulty rearing their children, and one or more are retarded, usually the retarded child is taken out of the home first, because the retarded have less adaptive ability and often more behavior problems than the normal children.

Ten-to-thirty-year follow-ups of graduates of special classes for the mildly mentally retarded indicate the married retarded do not have more children than other married couples. Those retarded who have children tend to have larger families than the nonretarded, but the average retarded parent has just under one child each, which is less than the average for nonretarded.

BIRTH CONTROL

The educable retarded, like other people, need to know that there are safe, reliable methods of preventing pregnancy. They also need to be helped to make a decision about whether to have children, when to have them, and how many. It should not just be assumed that they can or should come to a decision about this on their own (a common parental view), or that someone else should make the decision for them (a common professional view).

Some people think that the retarded should be sterilized to keep them from becoming a sexual problem, but sterilization of humans does not change sexual desire. The operations performed do not remove any parts; they simply cut the tubes which transport the eggs or sperm to the place where they can be fertilized, or fertilize. The operation is different from that used for cats, dogs, horses, and cattle. In these animals the ovaries and testes are removed and the animal is truly "neutered." A sterilized human is not neutered. He is still a man or a woman with all his sexual parts and the same sexual interests he would normally have.

Sterilization is, however, a desired means of birth control among some retarded. It is still the only reliable form of birth control for the male retardate and it is becoming easier to obtain. In areas where it is still difficult, the Human Betterment Association of America can assist in obtaining voluntary sterilization of a retarded person.

In California it is increasingly easier to obtain sterilization. In rare instances even hysterectomies are done with tubal ligation, on the grounds that if you are not going to be able to get pregnant, why bother to menstruate? A hysterectomy done without medical indication, simply because the parent wishes to avoid a "nuisance," is not good medical practice. If infertility and lack of menses are both desired, a large injection of progesterone will do the same thing more safely.

Sterilization should never be done without the informed consent of the retarded person, for legal as well as moral reasons. The legal reason is that anyone could sue on behalf of the retardate alleging that an injustice was done if the operation was performed against the retardate's will or without his knowledge. The outcome of such a suit is unknown, since no suits have as yet been brought to the courts.

The moral reason is simply a matter of being straight and honest with the retarded. Like other people, the retarded appreciate being dealt with fairly and squarely and they are likely to be more productive and cooperative if they are treated this way.

> Carol, an 18-year-old graduate of classes for the educable mentally retarded, went to a modeling course to improve her appearance and self-confidence. Her mother then became afraid Carol would get pregnant out of wedlock and arranged for a tubal ligation which was performed without Carol's knowledge. Carol was told the operation was an appendectomy.
>
> Later Carol married and wished she could have children. The marriage failed and Carol never again made a successful adjustment living at home. She preferred to live with a series of men who would support her for brief periods of time.

A retarded person often needs someone to provide reliable information. Once he has been tricked by parent or guardian, he can never again be sure if he is getting reliable or crooked information from them.

For retarded women, sterilization is only one of several feasible methods of birth control. Other methods are intra-uterine devices (the newer ones such as the Dalkon shield are often effective even in women who have never been pregnant), birth control pills (which have to be taken under some form of supervision in order to insure their regular intake), and the three-month birth control shots.* This latter method has been well-accepted by retarded women, as it is not permanent and therefore not as threatening as sterilization, and yet does not require remembering something daily. Names of physicians who are knowledgeable about this method can be obtained by contacting the local office of Planned Parenthood. The birth control shots are not widely used because the duration of sterility is not certain. There are also occasional side-effects which are disturbing to some women, such as sporadic bleeding. The shots sometimes prevent menstruation, but some women see this as a good thing.

As far as safety is concerned, the birth control pills (taken regularly) are the safest form of contraception so far available because they provide the surest birth control without the risk of surgery. The mortality of pregnancy is not often talked about. The death rate from pregnancy is ten times that of the birth control pill.

SEX EDUCATION PROGRAMS

Few school districts have organized family life education or sex education programs geared to the mentally retarded, even if there are good special education classes for the educable and trainable retarded. There are few marketed audiovisual aids appropriate for the mentally retarded.

Many parents are frightened by the thought of sex education for the mentally retarded. They think that the lack of questions about sex from their retarded child means that the child is not interested in finding out the secrets of reproduction and sexual love. Retarded children, like others, generally do not like to embarrass their parents and if they think their parents would feel like sinking through the floor if they asked for sex information, they refrain from asking.

If the retarded are to get appropriate family life guidance, it should begin long before puberty and, to be most effective, it

---

* Intramuscular progesterone is marketed as a hormone, not specifically for birth control.

should occur in the home. This ideal is often not available because of the ignorance or indifference of parents, and the schools can never substitute for effective parents. Any information given at school which is contrary to what the child sees or hears at home is likely to have little or no effect on the child. There is, however, some benefit in school-sponsored family life programs. Parents, fearing that their child might be taught the wrong thing, often make the effort to find out what is being taught and are then better equipped or more comfortable educating their child themselves.

Rules on Sexual Behavior

Any workshop or facility with a significant number of sexually mature mentally retarded persons needs to establish and publicize rules about sexual conduct. If this does not happen the "rules" are likely to change from day to day and from person to person. This is very confusing to the retarded person, to the staff, and to the parents or caretakers. The justification for establishing and publishing rules in workshops is the history of incidents of public kissing, petting, and sexual intercourse, which are upsetting to the normal persons who are in control and frightening to some of the parents and guardians of the retarded.

The fact that incidents have occurred which fall outside what is generally acceptable in a work or school situation means that the retarded have been insufficiently informed as to what sexual behavior is socially acceptable. Just because "normal" people in work or school situations do not need reminders on what is acceptable sexual behavior in public does not mean that the retarded do not need them. If there are limits or rules, they need to be well-publicized in order to be effective. They will be better publicized if the parent or guardian is informed as well as the retarded person.

Rules, to be real, need to have some consequences if broken. These consequences also need to be publicized to the retarded and their parents or guardians. Most workshops seem to need much support and encouragement in order to make, publicize, and enforce such rules. The alternative to sexual rules is recurrent "crises" which are probably more time consuming, and also destructive to the mental health of the persons whom the schools and workshops are trying to help.

SUMMARY

What is a successful sexual adjustment for the mentally retarded? A sexually well-adjusted mildly retarded adult will probably be self-supporting, marry, and have 0 to 2 children. A sexually well-adjusted mildly or severely retarded adult has significant social interaction with the opposite sex and enjoys intimacy with others without being taken advantage of. He masturbates in private on occasion unless he is fully satisfied by a loving sexual partner. A sexually well-adjusted profoundly retarded adult enjoys a close relationship with a parent or caretaker; this relationship is not a pretense by the caretaker just to earn money or a sacrifice by the parent or caretaker which excludes all other meaningful relationships.

At present a great many retarded persons do not have a successful sexual adjustment. If professionals can agree on a definition of good sexual adjustment like the one in the preceding paragraph, they can more successfully work together to help the retarded attain a satisfying sexual life. When this happens, the retarded will be happier, more productive, and better accepted into our society.

REFERENCES

1. Abelson, R. B. and Johnson, R. C.: Heterosexual and aggressive behavior among institutionalized retardates. *Ment Retard*, 7:28, 1969.
2. Bass, M. S.: Marriage for the mentally deficient. *Ment Retard*, 2:198, 1964.
3. Bass, M. S.: Marriage, parenthood, and prevention of pregnancy. *Am J Ment Defic*, 68:318, 1963.
4. Berne, Eric: *Sex in Human Loving*. New York, Simon and Schuster, 1970.
5. Biller, H. B. and Borstelmann, L. L.: Intellectual level and sex role development in mentally retarded children. *Am J Ment Defic*, 70:443, 1965.
6. Blacklidge, V. Y.: *Sexual Behavior of the Mentally Retarded*. San Leandro, Calif., Alameda County Mental Retardation Service, 1971.
7. Boök, J. A.: Fertility trends in some types of mental defects. *Eugen Quart*, 6:114, 1959.

8. Charles, D. C.: Adult adjustment of some deficient American children. *Am J Ment Defic*, 62:300, 1957.
9. Hammar, S. L. and Barnard, K. E.: The mentally retarded adolescent. *Pediatrics*, 38:845, 1966.
10. Hammar, S. L., Wright, L. S., and Jensen, D. L.: Sex education for the retarded adolescent. *Clin Ped*, 6:621, 1967.
11. Meyen, E. L.: Sex education for the mentally retarded. *Focus on Except Child*, 1:1, 1970.
12. Mickelson, P.: The feeble-minded parent, a study of 90 family cases. An attempt to isolate those factors associated with their successful and unsuccessful parenthood. *Am J Ment Defic*, 51:644, 1947.
13. Morgenstern, M.: Sex education for the retarded? *PCMR Message*, 21:10, 1969.
14. Peck, J. R. and Stephens, W. B.: The marriage of young adult male retardates. *Am J Ment Defic*, 69:818, 1965.
15. Project on Recreation and Fitness for the Mentally Retarded, AAHPER and Sex Information and Education Council of the United States: *A Resource Guide in Sex Education for the Mentally Retarded*, 1968.
16. Reed, E. W. and Reed, S. C.: *Mental Retardation: A Family Study*. Philadelphia, Pa., Saunders, 1965.
17. Roberts, J. A. F.: High grade mental deficiency in relation to differential fertility. *J Ment Sci*, 93:289, 1947.
18. Rutter, M., Graham, P., and Yule, W.: *A Neuropsychiatric Study in Childhood*. Philadelphia, Pa., J. B. Lippincott, 1970.
19. Shaw, C. H. and Wright, C. H.: The married mental defective, a follow-up study. *Lancet*, 1:273, 1960.
20. Tietze, C. and Johnson, B. S.: Observation on the fertility of patients discharged from Laconia State School, 1924-34. *Am J Ment Defic*, 54:551, 1950.

Chapter 15

MENTAL HEALTH IN A LARGE STATE HOSPITAL FOR THE MENTALLY RETARDED

IRVING R. STONE

FAIRVIEW State Hospital, located in Costa Mesa, California, forty miles from Los Angeles, is somewhat unique in that its more than 1,700 patients reside within a city and not separated from one. A busy thoroughfare passes by its doors, shopping centers and private residences are across the street, and restaurants are nearby. The city's municipal golf course surrounds the hospital on two sides and public schools, colleges, and the University of California at Irvine are but minutes away.

What has all this to do with mental health? One must spend some time working in or visiting the hospital to get the true impact on the patients. For example, they are not separated from the community but are a part of it. They are taken for walks by ward attendants to the shopping centers and make purchases for ward parties; they go to restaurants for special treats; they get to understand what city life is like; they see how people engage in one form of recreation and even learn some of the pleasures of engaging in chasing a golf ball. Being close to the community, civic and service clubs visit the hospital and provide parties for the patients and even take over the financial responsibility of improving wards through contributions of furniture, rugs, and television sets. The community constantly visits the hospital through the regularly scheduled tours, thus learning about the mentally retarded and dispelling any misconceptions. High schools and colleges bring their students for tours at frequent intervals as part of their psychology, social studies, child development, and home economics courses. In turn, these students become interested in the patients, returning as volunteers

212

and future employees. Some of the neighboring colleges require their psychology students to spend twenty or more hours each semester as volunteers.

Contrary to the expectation that this may cause disruption, the presence of these visitors and volunteers adds much to the lives of the patients. Their spectrum of life is broadened; changes in environment are constant, thus displacing the possible monotony of ward life; and there is an enrichment in being exposed to new individuals who work with them. They learn to adjust readily to new people, yet remaining within the framework of a stable surrounding of the ward and its staff. In one ward, for example, one boy serves as an official greeter and meets visitors with assurance and pleasure. Another enjoys walking toward visitors showing off his new ability to walk, whereas formerly he was confined to a wheelchair. On this same ward these patients, all physically handicapped as well as being moderately and severely retarded, have thirty minutes of time set aside each day for wrestling. They love the tumbling about on a large mat and vie with each other even though they cannot walk.

Ward parties, plays, and special programs are frequent activities in which the patients participate in planning and performing. Patients helped in completing a float which was entered in two local parades and on which they sit, dressed in costumes appropriate to the special occasion. At the school weekly assembly, programs are devoted to a particular event or holiday, displays or projects are prepared, and discussions focus on them. Thus, there is a central but ever-changing theme for class programs. The patients take delight in showing at the assembly what they have made. Songs pertaining to the assembly's theme are learned during the week and each class sings them as their part of the program.

Color does much to improve the mental health of patients. To replace the typical buff or green walls of the wards, colors that are warm and often vibrant have been used to create a more cheerful atmosphere. Ward personnel have taken on themselves, but with the consent of the administration, the task of painting scenes of woodlands, birds and Disney characters, seascapes, and monkeys climbing up colorful trees painted on posts. When the children awake in the morning they see not drab walls but things that appear lifelike and cheerful.

To modify the typical sterile austerity of a ward, many have been partitioned into small units, furniture more in keeping with the concept of normalization* have been secured, and even rugs now displace the appearance of some of the bare tiled floors. On one ward a patient sat down on the carpeted floor, ran his hand over the carpet, and said, "I did not know floors were soft." To carry the normalization concept a step further, this ward also has a small dog as part of its "unofficial" complement and the young patients love to sit and play with it.

The hospital's sheltered workshop provides another example of how mental health may be enhanced in a large hospital for the moderately and severely mentally retarded. As with most workshops, patients are given a pay envelope each Friday, the contents of which represent a portion of their earnings. This amount may be spent in any way they wish. The balance is placed in their accounts for such activities as the annual trip they all make in the company of hospital personnel. They go on the train, bus, or plane to another city, visit the attractions there such as the zoo, stay in a motel, eat meals in restaurants, and return to the hospital with eagerness to relate their experiences to others.

The annual performance of a circus on the grounds of the hospital provides great excitement and pleasure for the patients. The circus is provided through the retired circus performers' organization, with many excellent acts selected from those wintering in California donating their services. As at all circuses, free popcorn, candy, and other "goodies" are distributed.

Perhaps the greatest contribution to good mental health encompassing that of other patients and staff, is the infusion of spirit, teamwork, and interest which stems from the hospital's administration down to the workers on the lowest rung of the employee hierarchy. Motivation must be developed and perpetuated—it cannot be merely discussed and allowed to grow on its own without some reason for its existence. Motivation flourishes when results are achieved, when patients make satisfactory progress, and when realistic goals are set and attained.

* The mentally retarded should be provided as normal a life as possible.

Program organization is in itself a method of fostering good mental health. The specific needs of each patient are not only identified but the treatment provided is more readily individualized and progress recorded. Program administration is centralized and the talents of the many disciplines directed and focussed on specific needs of the patients. Review and evaluation of the needs thus becomes more meaningful and feasible.

Whenever changes take place in either administration or organizational structure of an institution, there is bound to be some apprehension on the part of the staff which may spill over to the patients. It is important, therefore, that tensions be reduced to a minimum. Only by sharing with personnel the rationale for the changes, the method to be employed, and the goals and objectives, can this be done. Such was the case at Fairview State Hospital when, through legislative decree, the state hospitals in California were edicted to change both administrative responsibilities and development of hospital programs in conformity with recognized patient needs. A task force of responsible staff members met for more than a year with the Medical Director, studying, planning, and proposing needed programs and their directors. After the reorganization program was adopted but before it was implemented, the Medical Director and a committee met with all departmental and ward personnel to explain the why, what, and how of the organization. Information regarding the programs was reported in the hospital's house organ and a "hot line" was opened to the assistant to the Medical Director for any staff member to use in determining the validity of any rumor regarding the reorganization.

The effects of these educational and hopefully "preventive" measures were evident by the ease with which the transition from departmental to program organization was achieved. Beyond the questioning and doubts of a few, ward personnel fitted readily into the newer concept and no adverse effects were noted in patient care or attitude. Had this not resulted, mental health, as reflected by anxiety, tension, outbursts, or even running away by patients, may have been adversely affected.

Weekly dances held for the patients in the hospital's auditorium add much to their enjoyment. Those without gross physical handicaps are never reticent about getting on the dance floor, whether with a partner or solo. The stimulation of the music and pulsation of the beat offer a means to dispel tensions and make for happy, vibrant boys and girls of all ages. Their gleeful applause at the end of each song reflects the degree to which their mental health is enhanced.

The wide difference between the psychological concept of seeing versus perceiving is most clearly indicated in our attitude toward patients and their abilities. Formerly we viewed the hospital as the point of last resort, where there was no other place for them, and where they would sit in wards watching television, hopefully without causing the staff too much trouble. As we used to say, "What can you expect from a mentally retarded person?"

We now view patients and the hospital differently; we saw them before but we did not perceive their potentials. Thus, our attitude was sadly lacking in reality. Hospitals must be less the storeroom and more of a training center, a place to develop each patient to the highest level of his potential. We must view each patient as someone to be studied and worked with. We must expect more than in the past. The patient who formerly sat quietly in the ward dayroom must be kept active, not for activity itself but because activity brings response. They should be given an opportunity to try, whether it be as obvious a need as walking or crawling, feeding himself, or taking part in workshop activities, creative pursuits in a classroom, or going about the grounds by himself. The patients we expected little from are now producing results far beyond our former expectations. As one person expressed it so aptly, "The patients have not changed; it is our attitude toward them that has changed." We now perceive them and not merely see them. The hospital is not the end for them but is a stopping point for meeting a specific need in their total development.

The satisfactions of the patients in their accomplishments are matched by those of the staff who work with them. Fairview State Hospital has adopted the principle of "let's see what we can do." The staff is unwilling to accept for themselves complacency and from the patients inactivity. Getting the patients involved requires planning by the staff but the results warrant it.

One ward staff decided that it was time to do a little more for their physically handicapped children. They worked after hours designing and making costumes for a special Christmas show, worked up a script, and coached the children in what they were to do. Some of the children had to be propped up against a background wall but carried through their assignments with satisfaction to all. One may well imagine the great pleasure of their parents as they saw their youngsters performing in a manner they never believed possible.

Mental health is an important factor to parents, too. Many experience feelings of guilt in sending their children to a state hospital. A number of parents involve themselves in the hospital's activities not from guilt feelings but because they accept continuing responsibility for their children. The parents' organization of the hospital provided prizes for the best decorated wards at Christmas and raised money to purchase a three-car "elephant train," called the "Jolly Trolley," pulled by a tractor-like vehicle. The Jolly Trolley takes the children from wards to the school or canteen, and on rides about the grounds. Wards make reservations for the use of the train. It is available seven days a week for the enjoyment and recreation of the patients.

From the foregoing, can we determine either what makes for good mental health or what good mental health really is in a large state hospital such as Fairview? Is there any single thread which seems to wind through the activities or programs described? It seems to me that there is not a single thread but a multitude of threads, each woven in such a way as to form a pattern.

There is the happiness of the patients expressed in how they look, how they perform, and how they express themselves. There is the activity of patients through meaningful and coordinated projects, all focussed on developing skills and modifying behavior. There is the determination and pursuit of goals for hospital programs, for patients, and for staff. There is a well-motivated staff which enjoys the challenge of working with severely retarded boys and girls and who experience satisfaction in seeing the fruits of their labors. There is a dedicated administrative organization which is willing to be innovative and resolute in following through with programs. There are administrators who make changes not for the sake of change but because they are willing to accept new techniques, new challenges, and reorganization when needed without regard to status factors. There are interested, cooperative, and sincere parents and relatives who recognize the efforts of the staff and are happy with the results obtained. These are signs of good mental health—for all.

REFERENCES

1. Bayes, Kenneth: *The Therapeutic Effect of Environment on Emotionally Disturbed and Mentally Abnormal Children.* London, England, author, 1967.
2. Jacobs, Angeline M.; Nichols, Daryl G., and Larsen, Judith K.: *Critical Behaviors in the Care of the Mentally Retarded. Vol. II: Behavior of Attendants.* Pittsburgh, Pa., American Institutes for Research, 1969.
3. Klaber, M. Michael: *Conference on Residential Care.* Hartford, Conn., University of Hartford Press, June, 1968.
4. Kugel, Robert B. and Wolfensberger, Wolf: *Changing Patterns in Residential Services for the Mentally Retarded.* Washington, D.C.: President's Committee on Mental Retardation, January, 1969.
5. President's Committee on Mental Retardation: *Residential Services for the Mentally Retarded—An Action Policy Proposal.* Washington, D.C., author, May, 1970.
6. Sarason, Seymour B. and Doris, John: *Psychological Problems in Mental Deficiency.* (4th ed.) New York, Harper and Row, 1969.
7. U.S. Department of Health, Education, and Welfare, Public Health Service: *Planning of Facilities for the Mentally Retarded.* Washington, D.C., author, November, 1964.

Chapter 16

A SYSTEMS APPROACH TO MENTAL RETARDATION

ARTHUR SEGAL

THE mentally retarded individual in the community is subject to thrusts that can increase his retardation, maintain a status quo, or encourage a facade of capability.

A clinical definition of mental retardation that is mutually agreed upon by professionals, and that is comprehendible to the nonprofessional has yet to be formulated. The semanticist struggling to confine this medical diagnosis to a clinical entity with comparable variables has a horrendous assignment and is probably doomed to either failure or to a syndrome that has shadowed parameters. The mental health professions have explained mental retardation as deviations from average intellectual functioning. However, there is lack of agreement as to how far below average the individual must be before he may be diagnosed as mentally retarded; indeed professionals disagree as to the meaning of intellectual functioning on particular subaverage levels.

The definition accepted by the American Association on Mental Deficiency refers to "subaverage general intellectual functioning which originates during the developmental period and is associated with impairment in adaptive behavior." The phraseology is nonspecific and creates images that are adaptable to a wide variation of individuals who may be brain-damaged, neurotic, schizophrenic, autistic, deaf, or who may have any one of several physical or psychiatric disabilities. The A.A.M.D. definition provides the child's developmental period as an etiological base for mental retardation. However, many professionals diagnose persons of latency age, teen-age, and even young adults as mentally retarded on the basis of subaverage test scores, or observations of impaired social functioning. In this manner professionals contribute to the dilution of what is at best a flimsy definition.

The struggle to define and categorize on a scientific level that which is not understood may be explained as man's attempts to define and to control his environment. It is axiomatic that knowledge of one's environment increases the possibility of successful social and vocational relationships. It follows that an understanding of the mentally retarded by the professional enhances his ability to assist him. Conversely, ignorance of the needs and abilities of the mentally retarded is fraught with danger. For ignorance leads to anxiety and is defended against by withdrawal from the object of anxiety. Accordingly, the professional who feels he is unable to understand the mentally retarded may as a consequence retreat from all attempts to assist this group of individuals.

Another possibility is that the professional will draw on available misinformation about the mentally retarded to validate his belief that they are unable to use mental health services. Still another possibility is that the professional will accept the mentally retarded for service with the condition that the individual exhibit behavioral characteristics that allegedly identify "mental retardation." Accordingly, if the professional believes the misinformation about mentally retarded individuals, and he accepts a mentally retarded individual in treatment, he will anticipate that his client will conform to his expectations. If the professional believes his client is unable to gain independence, he will help his client be a more comfortable child. If his client is an eighteen-year-old moderately retarded adolescent, the effect may be to limit the growth and development of this young adult.

A social systems approach to mental retardation poses the premise that mental retardation is a social concept as well as a medical diagnosis and that the concept and diagnosis are cognitively entwined in the minds of many laymen and professionals. The medical diagnosis draws on measurable relationships between a child's observed intellectual and social functioning, and normative functioning at age levels. The medical diagnosis defines the child's difficulty and may be used to prognosticate the child's growth potential in accordance with his level of retardation. The social concept of mental retardation is another matter. It is a symbol of ignorance, awkwardness, immaturity, and inability in man. The symbol embodies centuries of folklore; tales that have assumed facades of fact and that have found recognition in texts used to prepare students for the health fields. The mental retardation concept finds expression in the variations of arguments that espouse Darwinian themes of survival of the fittest and that justify maximum use of health, education, and welfare funds by individuals of "high moral fibre" and of "average to high" intellect. The etiology of this polemic is embedded in parental attitudes carefully nurtured over the child's early years; attitudes that teach the values of "smartness" and of "competitiveness," attitudes that seed ego ideals. The cycle finds structure in the social institutions that develop policies regarding which individuals will be served, and methodology defining how they will be served. The social institution provides a fertile field for the pollination of values that will respond to the nourishment provided by staff attitudes.

The concept of mental retardation is a set of beliefs pertaining to man's ability to function in social institutions. These notions have pervasively rippled over time and find expression on every level of community planning.

Mental retardation as a medical expression presents burdening obstacles to everyone called upon to live with it and to provide assistance to the identified individual. Mental retardation as a social concept frequently clouds the real medical syndrome and prognosis, and may in fact throw additional obstacles in the path of the disabled individual. For example, the child with Down's syndrome may not be taught independent living skills because supposedly "he will harm someone if he is out alone," or, "he does not need independence because he lacks emotional feelings for these things." On the other hand there may be a total absence of medical anomalies but behavioral expression suggests that the individual's conflict with school or job is a consequence of social and intellectual inability. It is then possible for this individual, in accordance with the mental retardation concept, to *become* "mentally retarded" and to be eligible for a system of services specifically designed for him; to be tolerated by systems designed for the general population—hospitals, recreation programs; and to be denied access to systems that insist they are unable to help the "mentally retarded."

An understanding of mental retardation and the necessary skill to provide mental health services to the so-labelled individual is derived from a stance that synthesizes medical, psychological, sociological, and anthropological knowledge. Figure 5 attempts to relate this knowledge to the mentally retarded individual and to suggest a mental retardation system.

The community mental health professional entering the mental retardation system must indeed pause to question where to start. The mental retardation system is a complex one and the variables

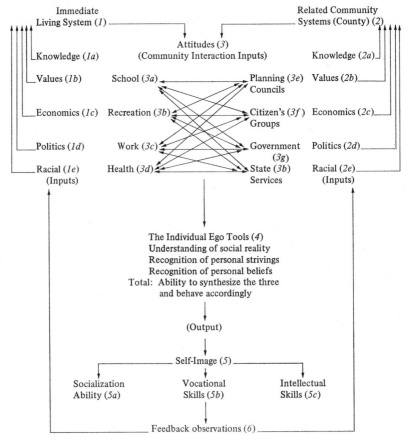

Figure 5. The mental retardation system.

contributing to what Perry[7] refers to as the "production of mental retardation" are many and difficult to treat by either education or circumvention. Careful analysis of the system is required in order to identify intervention points, to assess the system's tenacity, and to evaluate change potential for each of the units in the system.

1. Immediate Living System Center. The mentally retarded individual resides with his family or with parent surrogates. The parents' attitudes and beliefs about mental retardation are formed by the elements influencing the family, *(1a), (1b), (1c).* The attitudes may produce stereotypes about mental retardation that will influence the kind of education, recreation, vocational, and medical service they seek for their child and the expectations they hold for the outcome from the relationship with the service.

2. Related Community Systems. The mentally retarded individual dwells in a community of systems. This concept pushed to infinity includes the universe. For discussion in this chapter we will limit the community of systems to the county in which the retarded individual lives and caution the reader to be mindful of the larger systems (governments, professional organizations, research groups, etc.) that affect the defined community of systems. The county system is subject to a series of influences from the citizens *(2a), (2b), (2c),* and includes a multitude of organizational and family systems each influencing each other as well as the enclosing system. The resulting brew flows in the form of status, authority, and funding to the community organizations, some of which are listed under *(3).* Accordingly, the ability and desire of any one organization to serve the mentally retarded varies with its understanding of the problem and with its motivation in this area.

3. Community Interaction Inputs. The retarded individual's experience in any one organization is affected by the continuous interaction between these systems *(3a), (3b), (3c), (3d), (3e), (3f), (3g), (3h).* Interorganization relationships relating to case conferences regarding individuals or to coordinated social planning may raise or lower the level of service for a particular individual in one organization but not in another so that he may receive varying messages about himself.

4. The Individual Ego Tools. The ability of the mentally retarded individual to grow and to function in the community varies with: (a) his understanding of the messages he receives from his family and other community organizations; and (b) his manner of integrating these messages with his personal strivings and his personal values.

5. *Self-Image.* The individual's response to the messages he receives is in the form of a self-image that ranges from adequate role model to inadequate role model. The derivations of his self-image are observed in his ability to function at his capacity in social, vocational, and recreation activities.

6. *Feedback Observations.* The family and community observe the mentally retarded individual as he performs at activities. The nature of his performance influences the observer's attitudes and thus may perpetuate or alter the cycle.

RELATED COMMUNITY SYSTEMS

Mental retardation as a concept presents a social problem in that superimposed on a medical problem is a series of attitudes, fears, and false beliefs that tend to perpetuate and to exaggerate the individual's handicap. This community response (or it may be confined to a particular unit of the community) may in fact pose a seemingly impenetrable wall to intellectual and psychic growth in many of the retarded.

Attempts to use educational methodology to change attitudes may be thwarted if the interventions pose a threat to well-established values. For example, recreation or school units on the community level (Fig. 5, no. 3*a*, 3*b*) may express fear of retarded children even though they have scheduled special programs in response to community legal or moral persuasion. The fear expressed by the staff is embedded in tradition and probably would submerge arguments meant to calm it. Since staff attitudes have a direct bearing on staff expectations of the mentally retarded, and since staff expectations have a direct relationship to the child's ability to learn, it appears urgent that we find interventions that will induce change in staff attitudes and staff expectations. A professional who has inaccurate knowledge about mental retardation and who adheres to a Darwinian philosophy at a work training center tells of a month-long search to locate a dentist who would provide orthodentures for a moderately retarded young girl. The response of several dentists was that a mentally retarded girl has no need for nonessential treatment, and a few thought that the improvement of her appearance might lead to sexual activity!

The community system is a determinant of the delivery of service to a mentally retarded individual. The community system on a county level is complex. It allows for government groups, citizen groups, and associations of professionals to share beliefs regarding needed service and available resources. Applications for new programs are reviewed by these groups whose decisions support or find fault with the new proposal. A foster placement of mentally retarded adults may be blocked by the neighborhood housing association. The parent group for the mentally retarded may contribute data to the mental health advisory committee to support the need for new county positions in mental health programs serving emotionally disturbed adolescents who are in the educable mentally retarded class. If it were not for the representation from this group, the mental health advisory committee might allocate a higher priority to the requests of other groups of citizens and professionals.

Economic conditions affect the availability of jobs for the mentally retarded as well as the ability of county and private groups to fund new programs. Political movements alter treatment philosophies and it is possible that two different political activities may in fact be in conflict with each other to the detriment of service to the mentally retarded. The move in California to develop out-of-hospital residential placements for the mentally retarded along with expanded community mental health programs is accompanied on the county level by citizens refusing to vote the funds necessary for expanded community services for the retarded.

The many complex and interrelated factors that contribute energy to the community system have a direct bearing on the mental health of the mentally retarded. One obvious product of the county system is the service program for the mentally retarded. The size and quality of the products are determined by the priorities of the individuals who participate in the system and who shape the product. However, once the product is on the market it is the salesmen (agency staff) and the consumer (the mentally retarded and their families) who must live with it. This input to the mental retardation system is assigned slight significance by the professional, although I suspect the input has great effect on the mentally retarded. For instance, the social worker who recognizes the mental health needs of the mentally retarded individual but cannot help him may be initially challenged to identify an unknown program or to develop a new one. However, if the social worker is frustrated by the indifference of his superiors and by public apathy he may turn to professional pursuits that offer greater satisfaction. As a result he may visit his client less frequently or he may focus his visits on helping the client "adjust" to a less than adequate living environment.

The poignant message of rejection is keenly heard by the parents of the mentally retarded and by the moderately and mildly mentally retarded who are well aware of their exclusion from the mainstream of life. The mentally retarded are well aware that their participation in school, recreation, and job activities is on a track that runs parallel to the one used by their siblings and friends and that the track they take is not quite the same. The consequence of this self-awareness is reflected in the individual's image of himself and in the behavioral expressions he utilizes to express himself.

IMMEDIATE LIVING SYSTEM

The influence of family dynamics on the child's growth has been amply documented and these observations of parent-child dynamics may be dittoed in the family having a mentally retarded member. The family response to a mentally retarded child has been described in many publications. One response is the chronic grief[6] that parents suffer in the recognition of the reality of their child's disability. Other family responses may include feelings of anger and a desire to reject the child. The family may feel isolated from friends and may in turn respond by limiting their socialization with adults to others who also have a disabled child. The intensity of family dynamics is great and may engulf the novice practitioner who is misled by emotional facades and who fails to analyze the family as a group.

The response of individual family members to the mentally retarded member will fall along a continuum ranging from acceptance to rejection, from love to hate. The response is not static, indeed it wanders from end to end of the continuum, and any one response is relatively unimportant to the relationship between parents and child. It is the pattern of relationships between each of the family members that must be analyzed to determine the nature of the communication received by the mentally retarded member. The family is similar to formal organizations in that it has a structure with goals and norms governing relationships with other families and with the outside world.[1] The family is composed of members who in addition to their familial roles assume social roles that determine emotional relationships within the family as well as job assignments related to perpetuating the family. The mentally retarded child's security in the family has a greater relationship to his being able to enter into the family group without threatening its goals and the roles of other family members, than it has to a momentary emotional response between parent and child. His ability to enter school and later to work or to participate in a vocational workshop will be enhanced or hampered by his ability to participate as a constructive member in the family organization.

THE MENTALLY RETARDED INDIVIDUAL

A clinical analysis of the ego strengths and deficits of the mentally retarded individual is important to the mental retardation system. Knowing the influence of the immediate living system and the related community systems on the individual we seek information regarding his interpretation of these inputs and his ability to handle the data being fed through his relationships with family, peers, and agency staff. The individual's behavior is the visible data that describes his functions. Unfortunately the conclusion frequently drawn by the observer (the professional, the parent, and the lay citizen) is that the behavior itself is a symptom of mental retardation and is a firm indication of the individual's disability. However it is not accurate to assume a direct relationship between observed behavior and performance ability. It may be, of course, that a specific mentally retarded individual is performing to his capacity and is interpreting his environment in such a way that he is able to comfortably cope with it. In this instance the relationship between observed behavior and performance ability may be accurate.

However, the mentally retarded individual, like any individual, usually has difficulty understanding and coping with reality. Accordingly his behavior reflects his ability to understand his environment and to respond to the many social situations with which he must contend. The intensity of his personal strivings and values is a variable quality as it is with any individual, and it is accounted for by the factors influencing his emotional needs and social norms. In this regard, a strong influencing factor on the individual is his family, his peers, and the others in his social system. His behavior is not a reflection of mental retardation but is an indication of his learning over a period of years and a demonstration of his ability to relate this knowledge to his emotional needs and values in such a way that he successfully copes with social demands. Accordingly, a mental health analysis of the individual accounts for mental retardation as a factor that identifies a range of abilities and lack of abilities in areas of intellectual capability to deal with social situations. The analysis then searches to determine the information learned by the mentally retarded individual and the ego mechanisms he is employing to interpret this data. The relationship between data received by the individual and the nature of the response by the individual can then be related to a third factor: the individual's ability to respond differentially to the social scene. This is an exceedingly difficult evaluation to make. It should certainly not be related to mental retardation or even to levels of mental retardation.

An evaluation of the mentally retarded individual's ability to change, and of his ability to use psychotherapy, is arrived at only after many hours of discussion between the mental health professional and the mentally retarded individual. It is during this time (which may extend into months) that the clinician and the mentally retarded individual can explore the boundaries of reality and can test the ego strengths necessary for growth.

Carl is a 21-year-old mildly retarded epileptic young man who was trained for a position as a dishwasher and placed on a job. He lost the job after two weeks due to behavior described as defiant and immature. Upon closer observation we learned that Carl was quickly frustrated when faced with a new problem or when tired. At these times he responded in the manner described by his employer. Carl was placed on a second job where his experience was similar. This position was terminated after six days.

One response to Carl is to "close his case" and refer him to an activity program providing only social and recreational activities. However, Carl has the necessary vocational skills for the job. His inability can be understood only by interpretation of his behavior. The frustration may signal psychic inability to understand orders or to make decisions. A second ego dysfunction may be his recognized inability to achieve the job he wants compounded by his inability to handle the emotional feelings these strivings engender. On the other hand the behavior may symbolize Carl's response to being called "mentally retarded." Let us assume that Carl's family assigned him the role of incompetent, and frequently informed him of his inability by overprotecting him from possible danger. Carl received the message that affection and esteem are related to being a sick child. On the other hand, Carl's siblings, who were physically able and bright children, also received affection and esteem. This disturbed Carl who found himself in a bind of wanting to be like his siblings and wanting the security of his parents. His frustration on the job would insure his dependency on his parents by proving to them that he is truly incapable. In addition, his "incapability" would have the secondary emotional gain of evoking from his parents feelings of anger and pain and thereby satisfying his personal striving to hurt them. These clinical wanderings are endless and in this instance serve the purpose of illustrating two points: the mentally retarded individual is as complex as any individual; and the behavior of the mentally retarded individual may not reflect mental retardation but may represent a response to pressures from others.

John C. is a ten-year-old vibrant, freckled faced youngster who evidences minimal brain damage. He is the progeny of an Italian-American family residing in a large metropolis. The family income is moderate and achieved by the father's hard labor, an income threatened by the effects of inflation and the competition from newly arrived labor groups. Mrs. C. has a younger daughter who is very pretty and very bright. Mrs. C. enjoys her daughter's creativity. Mrs. C. frugally saves every penny, realizing that John will probably need funds for special assistance. She deprives herself and her family of little desserts in order to put away money for her son.

John entered school filled with a desire to learn and to have fun. His kindergarten teacher noticed unusual behavior in activities requiring fine motor control as well as some difficulty in expression of affect when relating to other children. A series of psychological examinations revealed that John had an "IQ of 60, minimal brain damage, and emotional upset diagnosed as a character disorder, manifested by a need to control and to manipulate games with other children." The school had no class for the educable mentally retarded (EMR) and John was ineligible for a class for the trainable mentally retarded (TMR). The school in the neighboring district had an EMR program but transportation difficulties prevented the use of that program. The school did have a federally financed program for underachievers and John was deemed eligible for that class. He remained in this class for two years. He continued to demonstrate difficulty in academic achievement, although his socialization skills profited by the relationship he had with tutors and small groups. After the second year he was reevaluated and found to have an IQ of 54. He was then placed in a class for the TMR, and at that time assumed the label "mentally retarded."

The school district had a progressive view of mental retardation although the principal of this particular school was locked in a struggle to develop manners and facades in her pupils at the expense of academic achievement. John's eagerness for activity combined with his fear of close peer relationships exposed him to the principal's personal beliefs about mental retardation: that they are defenseless children who need protection. Continued confrontations between John and the principal and several parent conferences evoked in John's family heightened feelings of shame and anger about John and their "upbringing" of the boy. The result was a state of family tension and misunderstanding.

*　　*　　*

Mary P. is an eighteen-year-old blond and a very pretty young lady. She resides in a foster home in a community of about 150,000 that provides bedroom space for a nearby bottling plant and several other small industrial operations. Mary is moderately retarded, IQ 48. She lived with her parents until twelve years ago when her parents divorced. Mr. P. disappeared and Mrs. P. placed Mary in a state institution in order to make a new life for herself. Mrs. P. is now remarried but fears Mary's presence in the home will disrupt the marriage. Mary completed school at the state institution one year ago and was then placed with the Johnsons, a hardworking family that includes seven other young adults who had been institutionalized.

While at the institution Mary developed some kitchen skills and maid skills. She has improved this past year with the Johnsons. In fact most of her time is used to exercise these skills. The remainder of her time goes into television viewing and leisurely strolls to the market where she handles simple purchasing of food.

Mary is friendly and relates casually to most of the people in the community. On occasion Mary is unsettled by thoughts of her mother and stepfather but appears to be easily "talked out of this" by the Johnsons who disclaim any reference to Mary experiencing emotional pain. They view Mary's expression as a reflection of curiosity that can be satisfied by simple explanations.

Mary attends church each Sunday and sings in the choir. Her participation in the choral group is profusely welcomed and her attendance strictly protected by lavish compliments, after which she remains isolated.

The task for the community mental health professional working with the mentally retarded is manifold. The two vignettes illustrate the complex lives of the mentally retarded in the community. The conflicts that surround John and Mary demand intervention at several points: the immediate living system, the related community system, the community interaction, the individual and the self-image (Fig. 5). A treatment plan should be developed in response to an assessment of the functioning of each of the elements of the mental retardation system as well as an evaluation of the interrelationships between the elements.

It is important to know the influence elements have on each other prior to directing treatment interventions at them. In other words it is necessary to view the mentally retarded individual from a position that recognizes the inputs from each element and that relates the individual's response to those systems. Only then is it possible to evaluate the psychodynamics operating in the mentally retarded individual. Only then, for instance, is it possible to distinguish between a distortion of reality, an inadequate attempt to cope with reality, and an inappropriate response to reality but one which is validated by the individual's family or teacher and is *ergo* the truth.

In terms of the mental retardation system (Fig. 5) a distortion of reality is at *(4)* and the intervention would be psychotherapy or group therapy; an inadequate attempt to cope with reality is at *(5)* and the intervention would be education in specific skill and feedback *(6)* to the immediate living and related community systems after the skill has been achieved. An inappropriate response to reality albeit one that is validated by the immediate living system *(1)* or the related community systems *(2)* is at *(1a), (1b), (1c), (1d), (1e),* and *(2a), (2b), (2c), (2d), (2e),* and the interventions would be family education and consultation with the community systems. However, a system requiring intervention at only one level is rare. Mental retardation is both a diagnosis of intellectual inability as well as a set of notions interpreting the diagnosis. The associated behavior syndrome has relationship to both the individual's deficiency in capability and to the subjective evaluations of those who relate to him. The consequence of this integration of fact and belief is observed in the ensuing relationships between the mentally retarded individual and others in the system.

Mary's case portrays the problems issuing from the foster parents' inability to separate fact from belief. They were aware Mary had limitations but they were blocked by personal belief *(1a)* from recognition of her strengths. As a result of their attitudes about mental retardation *(3)* they would not consider the use of a mental health center to assist Mary with her fears; nor would they venture to entertain thoughts about developing a semivocational future for Mary, such as an aide position in the community hospital, and participation in a nearby recreation program. A treatment plan that is responsive to Mary's mental retardation system would include interventions at *(1a)* and *(1b)* to allow Mary great opportunity for self-expression and to help the foster family plan a creative future with Mary; interventions at *(3)* to educate the minister and his choir about mental retardation in an effort to help them recognize Mary's strengths and to enjoy her company; intervention at *(3)* to encourage a vocational training program for Mary and at *(3c)* to develop a job placement in the community hospital; interventions at *(5)* to help Mary build new socialization and vocational skills; and interventions at *(4)* to help Mary cope with her past and to respond to the immediate living system and to the community interactions system as she experiences the attitudes expressed by her foster parents, the minister, and the choir.

A systems approach to John and his family first notes the inputs contributing to the boy's difficulties: family attitudes that stress hard work and self-sufficiency attitudes *(1b)* tinged by fear of inflation and of labor competition *(1c);* confusion at school about John's difficulty: an underachiever or a mentally retarded child *(3a);* the principal's personal beliefs about mental retardation *(3a).* We recognize that John's ego tools are weak *(4);* that he confuses his father's difficulties with his own and that he has difficulty controlling his personal strivings. The result is a fearful child who angers easily and socializes poorly with other children *(5a).* We are unaware if John has neurological deficits. The kindergarten teacher reported fine motor control difficulty but the school psychologist did not believe the request important and failed to seek a neurological evaluation.

The professional's interventions may be to change the inputs coming from the family *(1)* and from the school *(3a);* to strengthen John's ego tools *(4);* to help John gain new socialization skills *(5a);* and to refer John for a neurological evaluation. His selection of interventions may be guided by reality factors governing the availability of specific elements of the system to his intervention. He can move to help the family explore internal issues to plan for John and his sister. He probably cannot alter the principal's attitudes, however, he may be able to find help for John through the school district director of special education. Individual psychotherapy might threaten John because of his poor socialization ability. However, a tutor to provide individual instruction in both academic and leisure time activities might encourage John to experiment in relationships with peers. Consultation with the teacher would offer her the support needed to recognize John's strengths and to identify these for him and for his family.

CLOSURE

The mental retardation system is strengthened and protected by man's need to understand and to control his world; by his need to define as deviant behavior that which is dissimilar to his own and which is expressive of attitudes that threaten him. Thus

2 34   *Mental Health Services for Mentally Retarded*

the system is renewed with each observation of the mentally retarded individual's inability to perform at a task or to behave appropriately. Recognition of the system and assessment of its operation allows the community mental health professional treatment options that do not exist if therapy is confined within the treatment agency. Helping the mentally retarded individual and his family cope with the present and plan for the future is dependent upon treatment interventions in each part of the mental retardation system. The development of community mental health centers which join with other community agencies to offer an integrated educational and treatment approach is a step toward understanding that individual behavior is a consequence of a social system and that this system may be individualized for each person. It may be that the mental health agency that integrates its work with the community system will engage mental health generalists: professionals who are able to intervene on all levels of the system in behalf of his client in addition to the mental health specialist who because of his stance may be limited to treatment interventions in one element of the mental retardation system.

REFERENCES

1. Briar, Scott: The family as an organization: An approach to family diagnosis and treatment. *Soc Serv Rev*, 38:3, September, 1964.
2. Cohen, Nathan (Ed.): *Social Work and Social Problems:* National Association of Social Workers, 1964. See "Introduction" and "A Social Work Approach."
3. Dexter, Lewis A.: On the politics and sociology of stupidity in our society. In Becker, Howard (Ed.): *The Other Side: Perspectives on Deviance.* Glencoe, Illinois, Free Press, 1964.
4. Goffman, Erving: *Stigma: Notes on the Management of Spoiled Identity.* Englewood Cliffs, New Jersey, Prentice-Hall, 1963.
5. Merton, Robert K.: The self-fulfilling prophecy. In *Social Theory and Social Structure*, Rev. ed., Chap. XI, Glencoe, Illinois, Free Press, 1957.
6. Olshansky, Simon: Chronic sorrow: A response to having a mentally defective child. *Soc Case Work*, 43:4, April, 1962.
7. Perry, Stewart: Notes for a sociology of mental retardation. In Philips, Irving (Ed.): *Prevention and Treatment of Mental Retardation.* New York, Basic Books, Inc., 1966.
8. Segal, Arthur: Some observations about mentally retarded adolescents. *Children*, 14:6, November-December, 1967.

Chapter 17

COMMUNITY ORGANIZATION OF MENTAL HEALTH SERVICES FOR THE MENTALLY RETARDED

Leopold Lippman and Stanley Meyers

IN the early days, community organization of services involved removal from the community. There were "insane asylums," where the "demented" and the "feeble-minded" were thrown together, and that's what the "community" offered in the way of "mental health services."

It did not much matter, of course, because the lunatics, idiots, and imbeciles were somehow subhuman anyhow, and they really had no feelings to worry about, and in any case they—especially the Mongolian idiots, the cretins and such—had a short life expectancy . . . so why bother?

Later on, as society differentiated its residential services as between the mentally ill and the mentally retarded, and as efforts were made toward education and rehabilitation, institutional care remained in the medical model. It was still a requirement, in most states, that the administrative head of the institution be a physician, most often a psychiatrist, and that clinical services be seen as dominant. (The reality, to be sure, was that the daily contact and continuing responsibility for care was vested in line workers known as attendants, or cottage personnel, but the tables of organization showed the doctors, nurses, psychologists, and social workers in charge.) The superintendents, however, functioned principally as administrators, rather than as clinical practitioners, and so even the few professional persons available were not always in a position to use their special skills.

The first step in community organization of mental health services for the mentally retarded must be to accept the fact that most retarded persons can live in the community, and in fact can develop to a higher level of capability and self-sufficiency if they have access to the services and opportunities appropriate to their need. This first step the communities of the United States have begun to take in the past quarter-century, in response largely to the activities of organized parents and friends of the mentally retarded, through local and state groups and the National Association for Retarded Children, and in response to recommendations of the President's Panel on Mental Retardation.[6]

Nevertheless, as recently as the spring of 1970, Pennsylvania's commissioner of mental retardation said many people in his state "still want large warehouses for the mentally retarded." There is a great resistance on the part of many within the community to have the mentally retarded in the community at all, he said. He emphasized his own view that the community is the key to the development of appropriate and adequate services for the mentally retarded, both those who need residential services and those who are living at home; but he placed the blame for inhuman conditions in state school and hospital on the citizens who had paid little attention to the institutional situation until a scandal broke.

Acceptance of the retarded as individuals, and of their problems as legitimate concerns of the community, implies a concern for the retarded person as a member of a family. Community organization for mental health of the mentally retarded, therefore, properly starts with the needs of the total family. If the community does not address itself to the needs and feelings of the parents, in particular, it virtually guarantees the development of mental health problems for the retarded person and those around him.

Yet, even in quite recent times, the mental health implications of mental retardation have not always been clear, even to professional people. A mental retardation authority in New England requested permission to confer with the board of directors of a state mental health association in his region; and a few months later, he approached a metropolitan mental health association in a nearby community. In both cases, the answer was the same: "What does mental retardation have to do with mental health?" He never did receive an invitation to meet with either board.

The realities about mental retardation have changed. Antibiotics have extended the life expectancy; rehabilitation concepts have shown that it is possible for mentally retarded people to become self-reliant to a considerable extent—yet popular expectations remain much the same as two decades ago.

The most significant impact in recent years has come from two sources: the organization, and consequent pressure, of parents of the mentally retarded; and the interest of the White House, which began with President Kennedy and led to the work of the President's Panel on Mental Retardation.[13]

The parent groups began, in the 1930's and 1940's, as essentially PTA-type organizations in relation to the state institutions. Typically, they adopted such names as Children's Benevolent League (Washington) and Welfare League (New York). The organization of the National Association for Retarded Children, in 1950, represented a breakthrough, not the least important part of which was the open acknowledgement of retardation as a personal, family, and social problem, and a consequent challenge to all community agencies to find solutions.

The basic principles enunciated by the President's Panel on Mental Retardation gave further impetus in the same direction. The thematic concepts were as follows: there should be a continuum of services for the mentally retarded, to meet their changing needs throughout a lifetime; and insofar as possible, services should be provided close to home. These principles came as a striking alternative to the old pattern of "put him away and forget him" or "take him home and love him," neither of which saw the retarded individual as a human being with any potential, nor his family as anything but an object of pity.

Organizationally, it is interesting to note that in the United States the National Association for Retarded Children (NARC) developed quite independently of the National Association for Mental Health (NAMH), despite the occasional instances of cooperation and mutual assistance. In Portland, Oregon, for example, the local ARC received its genesis, encouragement and for a time even housing and staff support from the local AMH; but this was rare. At the national level, after more than a decade of separate existence with scant communication, a working agreement was developed between NARC and NAMH—but even the proposal for the president of each organization to sit ex officio on the other's board of directors was rejected by the mental health organization. In England, by contrast, the National Society for Mentally Handicapped Children received considerable impetus and continuing encouragement from the National Association for Mental Health; and the National Association for the Mentally Handicapped of Ireland includes scores of organizations in its constituency, many of them only tangentially concerned with mental retardation but recognizing it as a broad social problem.[4a]

The new community emphasis, growing from the efforts of NARC and the President's Panel on Mental Retardation, came to flower in the mid-1960's. Acceptance of a community responsibility for provision of services at the community level focused on the need for community organization as a newly applicable technique. In turn, creative professional people and program planners began to see the public residential facility (formerly known as "state institution") as part of the continuum of services, and hence as part of the pattern of community resources for the mentally retarded.[2] At this point—at least where the recognition was genuine rather than merely formalistic—the mental health resources of the residential facility were added to those of the community, to enrich the range of services available to the retarded person and his family.

What are the mental health problems associated with mental retardation? The images conveyed by two unusual books: *Flowers for Algernon*[4] and *The Cloak of Competence*,[3] suggest the dimensions of the problem. The truth is that the more mildly retarded an individual is, the more aware he is of his own difference from others.

Because the citizen movement for the mentally retarded started with parents, the first emphasis was on the needs of retarded children. As the retarded grew older, the perception remained one of a childlike quality, rather than of a retarded person growing to adulthood. By contrast, in the field of mental illness, except for child guidance clinics, the providers of service and society for the most part visualized the mentally ill and disturbed as adults.

When a family receives a diagnosis of mental retardation, particularly in early childhood, a series of agonizing questions immediately come to mind: What do we tell the grandparents? How do we explain to our other children? What does mother tell her girl friends? How do we deal with the baby shower? Does the family have open house and invite the friends and neighbors to see the baby? What does one put on the birth announcement? Do we take the child for a stroll in the carriage? What do we tell the neighbors? How do we handle their questions, their stares, their avoidance?

Guilt . . . shame . . . denial . . . rejection. . . . All the natural reactions of shocked and ego-traumatized parents are likely to be negative. If the marital relationship was weak, immature, or shaky to begin with, it is further threatened by such an experience. If the professional (usually the obstetrician or pediatrician) does not deal skillfully and immediately with the desperate need for counseling, the parents' fears and negative reactions are reinforced.

To cope with this universal problem, local associations for retarded children throughout the United States have given the support of the organized parents to the "new" parents who otherwise would have felt alone with their problem. More, the local associations have often established counseling or group therapy mechanisms to help the parents over the first shock. The Tacoma-Pierce County Chapter of the Washington Association for Retarded Children, for example, for several years in the 1950's and 1960's sponsored a monthly Parent Education Clinic, to which "new" parents were invited and at which a variety of professional people (doctors, psychologists, social workers, teachers) spoke and answered questions. Each parent (or couple) attended as long as he felt the need, and he then found his way to the services he or his family required.

The responsibility for family counseling ought not to rest, however, solely with the parent organizations. Enlightened social agency executives in some communities have developed similar services under professional auspices, as part of their service to the community at large, including parents troubled by a variety of family problems. The birth or diagnosis of a mentally retarded child may trigger a family crisis, or it may exacerbate problems already in existence, but in either case the generic social agency has a responsibility to meet the emotional needs of the whole family.[1a]

Traditionally, the "family" of the retarded person is seen as the parents. In truth, the family embraces a good many other people, all of whom have mental health pressures and needs of their own: the grandparents (think of them also as in-laws), the siblings (especially, but not only, the adolescent sisters), the nubile sisters and cousins of the retarded child's mother (troubled by genetic implications), the girlfriends and the boyfriends and the neighbors . . . all of whom see the newly-labelled "retardate" in terms of their preconceptions and often in a framework of mis-information. Each of these individuals, in turn, may by his thought-less reaction further contribute to the misery, guilt, and rejection of the parents. One grandfather comes to mind, whose rejection of his own son on the birth of the retarded grandchild was so austere and so complete as to blight the lives of the entire family forevermore, and to drive the parents and the child into mentally unhealthy paths of action from which, ultimately, they could not retreat.

In the past decade, an increasing number of states have under-taken formal approaches to organization of community services for the mentally retarded. The leaders, for the most part, have developed regional mechanisms, as an intermediate and workable level between state government and the localities.

In Connecticut, for example, which was one of the first, the state has been divided into twelve regions, each with a popula-tion of approximately 400,000. The regional center, which pro-vides residential services for an average of one hundred retarded children and adults, also offers specialized services not only for the residents but for up to 250 retarded persons in the nearby communities who can benefit from such services on a day basis. Wherever possible, however, the personnel of the regional center stimulate existing community resources to provide locally-based services for retarded persons. The regional center then serves as a back-up resource as well as a residential facility for short or long-term care as the individual circumstances may require. The state of Connecticut has come to assume the basic responsibility, financial and administrative, for residential services and day care.

The keynote of the Connecticut program is flexibility and responsiveness to the individual needs of the retarded person and his family. Each of the twelve regional programs carries the responsibility of serving all retarded persons in its area. Voluntary agencies are eligible for grants-in-aid to provide day training, diagnostic service, and/or vocational training. Where children of school age are in residence in a regional center, the local school system provides classes in the public school. Buses pick up and return children to the center each day.

Regional centers will provide residential service for one day and up. Families can place a retarded child for emergencies, for vacation, for lack of a baby-sitter, or other reasons.

In addition, the regional centers have opened foster homes, providing back-up to the foster families with short-term residence in the center as required as well as activities for the retarded individual outside the foster home. In one case a forty-five-year-old woman, mildly retarded with no living relatives, was referred for placement. Instead, a regional center took over the home in which she lived, placed two women of about her age, and employed staff to manage the facility. The cost was supplied by the woman's estate.

The regional program has come to be the fulcrum around which all services for the retarded and his family can be obtained or provided.[9]

In California, the same label—regional center—refers to quite a different organizational pattern. On recommendation of the Study Commission on Mental Retardation,[8] the Legislature in 1965[7] launched a program, which has now grown to statewide network proportions, whereby the State Department of Public Health enters into contracts with public or nonprofit agencies to provide diagnosis and counseling to retarded persons and their families through the regional centers. In addition, for those retarded persons who would otherwise require care in a state hospital, the regional center is authorized to find and to pay for alternative services, of whatever sort, which would meet the needs of the individual and his family. The scope of coverage is thus quite broad;

indeed, the law was amended in 1968 to provide for a state program of guardianship-protectorship, which is also being administered by the regional centers.[12]

A separate program, which originated considerably earlier, deals increasingly with the mental health needs of the mentally retarded in California. The Short-Doyle program, enacted in its original form in 1957, provides that county government, largely with state funds, may provide a wide range of mental health services to all its citizens, including the mentally retarded and their families. The law and the funding arrangements have been increasingly liberalized in recent years; and with the enactment of the monumental Lanterman bills of 1968 and 1969, the provision of mental health services at the county and state-hospital levels are now being integrated into a unified and coherent pattern. The State of California now undertakes to pay 90 per cent of the cost of mental health services, whether provided at the county or state level, and the county of residence of the individual is obligated to pay the other 10 per cent. The objective of this new pattern of organization is to insure that the individual receives the services he needs, in the setting most appropriate to his situation, rather than in response to financial incentives to hospitalize a person who might be better served in another way. The Short-Doyle program originated and developed over the first decade largely in relation to mentally ill and emotionally disturbed persons, and in some counties the mentally retarded were denied Short-Doyle services even when they had specific mental health needs. This has begun to change, however, as the county programs not only are coming to accept retarded persons who need psychiatric services, but are also reaching out to provide specialized services to the retarded as such.

Since 1954 in New York State, there has been a Community Mental Health Services Act, which makes state funds available in partial payment for local mental health services. There are differences between the New York law and the Short-Doyle program in California. For one thing, the local provider of service in New York may be a voluntary agency, although the contractual and fiscal arrangements always involve a local public agency, in an intricate arrangement of budgeting and bookkeeping. For another, the New York state payment represents a reimbursement of funds expended by the local provider, rather than a shared-funding or matching arrangement. Most important, however, the New York law has from the beginning embraced services to the mentally retarded among those covered by the "mental health" law, and although in the past the expenditures have been largely weighted in the direction of clinical services for the mentally ill and the emotionally disturbed, the state and many of the local agencies in the past few years have begun to adjust the balance to deal more equitably with the needs of the retarded. Responsibility for planning and stimulating services at the local level rests with the Community Mental Health Board (in New York City, reorganized and renamed the Department of Mental Health and Mental Retardation Services in 1969).

The New York State Department of Mental Hygiene, which administers the Community Mental Health Services Act through its Division of Local Services, involves itself in the provision of local services to the retarded through another channel as well. The Division of Mental Retardation, which originally had responsibility solely for the state schools for the mentally retarded, now has jurisdiction also over the hostel program, by which the state participates with local voluntary agencies in the development of community residential services for retarded adults who hold jobs and who otherwise can function in the community, but who require supervised living arrangements.

The Division of Mental Retardation also makes direct grants, up to 100 per cent of the cost of programs, to local service agencies for short-term specialized projects. One grant, for example, pays for homemaker service for families with severely retarded young children. Such children, who in the past would have been placed in state residential facilities at birth or shortly afterward, now may remain at home through early childhood, with assistance and relief for the mother.

New York City, although it is part of New York State and is subject to state laws and budgetary restrictions, is in many ways unique. Its population exceeds that of many states. Its annual expense budget is second only to that of the Federal Government. It is a national city, in that many of its economic, social, and health problems originate elsewhere, though they may come to New York for solution. People burdened with poverty, illness, inadequate education, cultural maladjustment, and many varieties of mental ill-health seek out the big city. Not only mental retardation which is organically based, but the subnormal functioning which originates in environmental deprivation, are to be found in high numbers in New York. The city is in many ways like a populous, yet problem-ridden state, but it does not have the resources or the powers of a state.

Nevertheless, the Mayor's Committee on Mental Retardation[1] following upon the New York State Planning Committee on Mental Disorders[10] and the President's Panel on Mental Retardation[6] recommended the development of regional programs, to stimulate the development and then to promote the coordination of mental retardation services on a community level smaller than the entire metropolis. The City Department of Mental Health and Mental Retardation Services has itemized eight areas of program service which the Mental Retardation Regional Programs, through councils of citizens and agencies, are now ordering into a priority sequence. The program areas are the following:

1. Prevention.
2. Early identification, diagnosis and evaluation, counseling for family, program placement for the child, and follow-up.
3. Day training.
4. Home care.
5. Public school classes.
6. Recreation and social programs.
7. Vocational training, sheltered shops, job placement, and follow-up.
8. Residential services.

The New York City approach to priorities of service recognizes that in each of the service areas there are sub-areas of need. Transportation, personnel recruitment and training, religious services, and dental services are examples. Of critical importance is the need for a *continuum,* to be achieved through a complex of services providing care and training to the retarded individual and his family, though not necessarily in one place.

In response to another recommendation of the Mayor's Committee on Mental Retardation, Mayor Lindsay in 1968 established the New York City Office of Mental Retardation. This small unit is essentially a community organization mechanism, its area of operation being principally within the municipal government. There has been organized an Interdepartmental Conference on Mental Retardation, through which representatives of some twenty departments and agencies of City government exchange information and develop cooperative working relationships. The Office of Mental Retardation works with municipal hospitals to develop diagnostic casefinding and counseling services; helps to train social service and other professional personnel in various departments; produces resource materials; promotes cooperation between public and voluntary agencies; and maintains liaison with Federal, State, and community agencies.

The development of community mental health centers, in response to Federal impetus which originated in the Kennedy administration, is in some parts of the nation beginning to deal with mental retardation as a mental health problem. The *New York Times* a year or so ago, in a half-page article with pictures, told of such a center in Brooklyn, New York, where a walk-in service is described as "storefront psychiatry." The identifying signs, and the staff, address the people in English, Spanish, and Yiddish; and this is the beginning of relating to the people's needs at their own level. As the psychiatrist who directs the program put it, "Whether the problem is drugs, rats, reading, or retardation, it is important to have a place to turn for assistance."

Not long ago, a Federal grant for staffing of new programs in mental retardation was awarded to a psychoanalytically oriented agency in the Northeast. As recently as June, 1970, a knowledgeable official commented that this was the first proposal funded under this program to provide mental health services for mildly retarded adults and their families.

In Colorado, the Division of Mental Retardation in the Department of Institutions has long and traditionally had responsibility for operation of the state residential facilities for the mentally retarded. In recent years, however, it has also encouraged and helped finance the development of regional and local programs throughout the state. The division has begun to organize its staff of social workers, so that none of them considers himself an exclusive employee of the state institution or of the regional or community program. Now they are employees of the division, at the state level, and they are free to give their professional skills to the retarded individual wherever in Colorado he may be. In some respects, this is similar to the provision of professional services to the retarded under national auspices in Denmark, where the physician, educator, or social worker may have a residential facility as his base of operations, but he serves retarded persons living at home or in other residential facilities throughout the surrounding area.

As programs proliferate, it becomes increasingly important to provide training for the personnel who will work with the mentally retarded and their families. Increasingly, the planners and directors of programs are recognizing that not every service worker must have full professional training; indeed, persons at subprofessional and lower skill levels may have a great deal to contribute, and may in some cases be more sensitive and responsive to the needs of the retarded than are some highly trained specialists. What *is* essential, to deal effectively with the mental health needs of the mentally retarded, is a) to recognize them as people, with human needs and some potential for development and b) to see them as part of a social construct, and most particularly as part of a family.

Beyond individual services to meet the needs of the retarded and their families, and beyond group therapy activities, recreational programs, supervised living arrangements and job opportunities, there is a larger setting in which society can create an atmosphere conducive to mental health for the mentally retarded. Public relations, defined in its broadest sense as effective human relations, can be a substantial positive force for mental health.

A continuing objective, to which the National Association for Retarded Children addressed itself from its organizing days around 1950, is the development of public awareness, public understanding, and public acceptance.[5] The task is not yet done, as numerous opinion and attitude studies in various parts of the United States show. It is easy to overlook the fact that even parents of retarded children were part of the "general public" before their children were diagnosed and labelled. If public opinion considers the retarded person inferior, and somehow less worthy of attention, concern and service, the "new parent," sharing this widespread attitude, starts to deal with his problem in an aura of ambivalence, guilt, and hopelessness. If, by contrast, society moves toward the acceptance of retarded children and adults as a social reality, the parents and the retarded individual start with hope and the prospect of success in making the best of their limited resources.

Creative public relations may express itself in many ways. In the State of Washington, one expression came, more than a decade ago, with the establishment of the first state school for the mentally retarded to be located on the edge of a major city. The residential facility was on a site less than a mile from the Seattle city limits, and a scant twenty-minute drive from the campus of the University of Washington. Added to the advantages of this proximity—which encouraged parents, professional people and the surrounding community to consider the institution open to them—there was a genuine and deliberate openness in the attitude and policies of the administration. The superintendent and his colleagues actively sought out community participation. As a result, hundreds of volunteers (ranging in age from senior citizens to high school students) gave thousands of hours of service and loving attention to the residents of the state school for the retarded. Even the impact on the state legislature was discernible; but more important was the direct and positive effect on the residents themselves.[11]

As mental retardation is recognized as a social challenge, and not merely a personal or family problem, the solutions will come more quickly. Among the happy results will be emotional tranquillity for the parents and self-respect for the retarded persons themselves.

And these are the elements of mental health.

REFERENCES

1. Adams, M.: *Mental Retardation and Its Social Dimensions*. New York, Columbia University Press, 1971.
1a. City of New York: *Report from the Mayor's Committee on Mental Retardation*. New York, 1968.

248   *Mental Health Services for Mentally Retarded*

2. Dybwad, G.: Community Organization for the Mentally Retarded. National Conference on Social Welfare: *Community Organization 1959.* New York, Columbia University Press, 1959.
3. Edgerton, R. B.: *The Cloak of Competence.* Berkeley, Calif., University of California Press, 1967.
4. Keyes, D.: *Flowers for Algernon.* New York, Harcourt, Brace and World, 1966.
4a. Lippman, L.: *Attitudes Toward the Handicapped: A Comparison Between Europe and the United States.* Springfield, Thomas, 1972.
5. National Association for Retarded Children: *Decade of Decision.* New York, 1959.
6. President's Panel on Mental Retardation: *A Proposed Program for National Action to Combat Mental Retardation.* Washington, D.C., Government Printing Office, 1962
7. State of California, Assembly Interim Committee on Ways and Means: *A Redefinition of State Responsibility for California's Mentally Retarded.* Sacramento, Calif., 1965.
8. State of California, Study Commission on Mental Retardation: *The Undeveloped Resource: A Plan for the Mentally Retarded of California.* Sacramento, Calif., 1965
9. State of Connecticut, Department of Health, Office of Mental Retardation: *One Low and Flickering Flame.* Hartford, Connecticut.
10. State of New York, Planning Committee on Mental Disorders: *A Plan for a Comprehensive Mental Health and Mental Retardation Program for New York State.* Albany, N.Y., Volumes I-VII, 1965.
11. State of Washington, Subcommittee on Mental Retardation, Governor's Inter-Agency Committee on Health, Education, and Welfare Programs: *Everybody's Child: The Mentally Retarded.* Olympia, Wash., 1961.
12. United Cerebral Palsy Associations: *Conference on Protective Supervision and Services for the Handicapped, Proceedings.* New York, 1966.
13. Wortis, J. (Ed.): *Mental Retardation: An Annual Review, I.* New York, Grune and Stratton, 1970. See Dybwad, G. and Dybwad, R. F.: Community Organization: Foreign Countries (pp. 224-238), and Lippman, L.: Community Organization: U.S.A. (pp. 239-249).

Chapter 18

TRAINING IN DELIVERY OF MENTAL HEALTH SERVICES FOR THE MENTALLY RETARDED

Elias Katz

THE previous chapters in this book have addressed themselves to such questions as: "Who are the mentally retarded?" "What mental health services do they and their families need?" "How can they be helped?"

The present concluding chapter is concerned with: "What training can be provided for professionals who are concerned with the delivery of mental health services to the mentally retarded?"

NEED FOR TRAINING

An acute and chronic shortage exists for trained personnel and technical help. Skills, knowledge, and attitudes about the retarded learned during the course of professional training often require modification or supplementation. New operational, clinical, and educational developments lag behind their general application in the field. It is necessary to provide training for those who are or will be responsible for planning, implementation, administration, and evaluation of mental health services.

Many possible approaches to training exist depending on the goal, as well as on the personnel to be trained. The basic aim of the mental health effort on behalf of the mentally retarded is to develop, maintain, and restore their social and personal equilibrium despite emotional stress. The training mission is to develop the necessary trained manpower to achieve the goal. The follow-

Note: The content of this chapter does not necessarily reflect the policies or procedures of the California Department of Mental Hygiene or of the Center for Training in Community Psychiatry and Mental Health Administration at Berkeley.

ing describes one approach which was used* at the Center for Training in Community Psychiatry and Mental Health Administration at Berkeley (hereafter called the Center). Starting in 1969, a sequence of four quarterly courses in "Community Mental Health Services for the Mentally Retarded" was offered at the Center. Since these mental retardation courses were unique, and were presented in the context of a unique community mental health training program, a brief overview of the Center's training program is in order.

THE CENTER'S TRAINING PROGRAM

The general objective of the Center's training program was to develop the principles, methods, and criteria for the practice and teaching of community psychiatry and mental health administration.[1] The curriculum consisted of four courses offered sequentially throughout the year in research as applied to community psychiatry, preventive services such as mental health consultation, administration of community mental health services, comprehensive community mental health services for the mentally retarded, and mental health services for children and youth in crisis.

The preventive, administrative, and research aspects of community mental health were taught as complementary or supplementary to clinical services in community mental health programs.[†] Not only was the faculty multidisciplinary, but mental health professionals of different disciplines were taught together. Supervised field work was provided in selected community mental health programs.

TRAINING IN MENTAL RETARDATION

The objectives[‡] of the Center's training in mental retardation during this period were the following:

1. To increase each trainee's skills:
   a. Formulating goals and objectives in providing treatment and supportive services for the mentally retarded.

---

* Between 1969 and 1971. Since 1971 there have been changes in the Center's operation.

† Clinical training was not provided at the Center.

‡ These objectives were periodically reviewed and adjusted in the light of Center staff, trainee, and agency interactions.

    b. Defining and solving problems arising in the course of the trainee's field work.

    c. Evaluating one's own and/or others' treatment and supportive services on behalf of the mentally retarded.

2. To increase each trainee's knowledge of the following:

    a. Current issues in prevention of mental retardation and in prevention of mental breakdown among the mentally retarded.

    b. Goals and objectives in providing care, treatment, and supportive services.[2]

    c. Various models and community resources for delivery of mental health services to the mentally retarded.

    d. Methods of providing treatment and supportive services for the mentally retarded.

    e. Evaluation of the effectiveness of mental retardation programs.

3. To act as a resource for information and expertise in delivery of mental health services for the mentally retarded.

The organization of course work used the Center's model of training: a blend of various elements—related supervised practice in selected programs providing mental health services to the mentally retarded and their families, tutoring by preceptors, weekly reading seminars, and a coordinated series of lecture-seminars.

Enrollment was open to qualified professionals working with the mentally retarded, including psychiatrists, clinical and school psychologists, social workers, nurses, rehabilitation counselors, physicians, and educators of the mentally retarded.

Field Work

Each trainee engaged in field work, which usually took the form of defining and working through urgent problems faced by the trainee in his work with the mentally retarded and their families. The field work was intended not only to be a learning experience, but an activity of practical value to the trainee and his agency.

Field work was approved by the trainee's supervisor. This meant that the trainee arrived at an understanding with his agency so that his field work would be consistent with the agency's goals and methods and would improve his knowledge and practice.

Examples of Field Work of Trainees

For her field work, a psychiatric social worker organized a weekly "Creative Living Program" for mentally retarded recipients of Aid to the Needy Disabled. The clients either came on their own or were brought to the program. They participated in games, social activities, and group discussions. For many, this was the only break from a very lonely and dull living experience. Efforts were being made to increase the number of days per week for the program.

A clinical psychologist was given major responsibility for training ward personnel in a program serving severely mentally retarded patients in a state hospital. His field work consisted of preparing two manuals for ward personnel, *A Method for the Evaluation of Self-Help Training for the Mentally Retarded, and Operant Conditioning as Self-Help Training for the Mentally Retarded.* These later became basic texts for use of ward personnel in instituting a behavior modification program for patients.

A clinical psychologist employed in a county mental health program made an extensive study of her own psychotherapeutic interventions with emotionally disturbed mildly retarded children in a public school. She documented many problems not only in dealing with the children but with the school administrators and teachers.

Tutoring by Preceptors

From two to four trainees met weekly with their assigned preceptor, who had been selected on the basis of training and experience in mental health services for the retarded. Previous experience at the Center had indicated that two or more trainees at a time appeared to accelerate the learning process through the free exchange of ideas and experiences. Many trainees shared new ideas, skills, and insights with their colleagues in their agencies or introduced to their communities a service, activity, or procedure that was overlooked or unrecognized.

Reading Seminars

Each week all trainees met with a faculty member in a reading seminar. Trainees discussed readings from textbooks, journals or reports, in preparation for the lecture of the day. There was also a discussion of the previous week's lecture. The Center provided an excellent library of publications in community mental health and mental retardation.

As in other Center offerings it was possible to assemble a distinguished faculty to present the lecture-seminars in the mental retardation courses (see Appendix).

THE MENTAL RETARDATION COURSES

Following are brief summaries of the objectives and content of each course in the mental retardation sequence.

Community Mental Health Services for the Mentally Retarded
(Summer, two weeks, full-time)

The general purpose of the first course in the sequence was to introduce the trainee to basic concepts of direct and indirect mental health services to the mentally retarded. This was followed by descriptions of agencies providing mental health services to the mentally retarded, including state hospitals for the mentally retarded, community mental health services, regional centers for the mentally retarded, state and county welfare agencies. Field visits were made to mental retardation programs.

Professional Approaches to Mental Health Services for the Retarded
(Fall, weekly, 1-6 PM, Fridays)

This course presented some of the approaches being used in providing mental health services for the retarded, with emphasis on different professional roles. It also included discussion of direct and indirect services such as psychotherapy, behavior modification, and mental health consultation. Weekly sessions were held with a preceptor to discuss field work, as well as weekly reading seminars.

Agency Approaches to Mental Health
Services for the Retarded
(Winter, weekly, 1-6 PM, Fridays)

This course was concerned with how different agencies deliver mental health services to the retarded. Emphasis was placed on the agency's objectives. Field work was discussed in groups with preceptors, and reading seminars were held weekly.

Recent Developments in Mental Health
Services for the Retarded
Spring, weekly, 1-6 PM, Fridays)

This was the final course in the sequence focussed on recent developments. Among the topics were sex education for the retarded, creative art expression for the mentally retarded, paraprofessional training, and the "Six-Hour Retarded Child." Trainees concluded their field work, writing up their evaluation of the experience, its impact on their colleagues, and its effects on the retarded they served.

Participants

During the two-year period covered by this report, some 140 trainees attended. A majority of the participants were psychiatric social workers, with smaller numbers of clinical psychologists, nurses, social workers, physicians, rehabilitation counselors, and teachers.

IMPACT OF THE CENTER'S MENTAL RETARDATION TRAINING PROGRAM

Some flavor of the impact of the Center's mental retardation training program during this period can be assessed on the basis of material from two sources: a) trainees' comments reported at the completion of each quarterly course, and b) the writer's impressions based on planning and conducting the courses, and interaction with Center faculty, trainees, and colleagues in the field.

Trainees' Evaluations of Course Work

At the conclusion of each quarter, trainees completed a questionnaire evaluating the quarter's course work. One of the questions was "In what ways do you think this training experience might prove to have benefitted you personally, as related to your job performance?" Following are some of the statements made by trainees:

> I feel encouraged—more confidence—feel less defensive about my special interest, less as though I'd taken them on by default. (Psychiatric social worker coordinating mental retardation services in a community mental health center.)

> It has given me a broader base of knowledge—interaction with the other disciplines has helped me—I will be more helpful to social workers now that I understand their functions—also other workers in the field. (Psychiatric nurse in state mental retardation hospital.)

> Better conceptualization of role of social worker in public assistance in integrating services to retarded. Emboldened to push for improved evaluation procedures at social worker level and at program level. (Social worker coordinating services for mentally retarded clients of a county welfare department.)

> Emphasis on importance of individualizing clients and working past, and forgetting the label of mental retardation. . . . (Psychiatric social worker serving mentally ill and mentally retarded patients on leave from state hospitals.)

> This experience has made me more aware of possibilities available to the mentally retarded, even those profoundly retarded, such as those on my ward. . . . I think this experience will help me form a more concrete treatment goal for each patient and a more concrete program. (Occupational therapist in state mental retardation hospital.)

> 1. It has given me information of programs of agencies with which we work.
> 2. It has exposed me to program which could be profitably duplicated in our area.
> 3. I have a desire to know more. (Psychiatric social worker serving mentally retarded patients on leave from state hospitals.)

> I enjoyed meeting the people and talking with them about their job or facility. Being new in the field I found this very beneficial. (Music therapist in state mental retardation hospital.)

> Because presently I am working with the severely and profoundly retarded in nursing homes, there was very little in this training experience which can be utilized by me on the job. However, as my assignment will change eventually, I may be expected to draw upon

my experiences gained through the Center. . . . (Psychiatric social worker serving mentally retarded patients on leave from state hospitals.)

Misconceptions, misinformation, and stereotypes went by the board. Where I came in with very clear ideas about mental retardation I leave with a broader understanding of the multifactorial syndrome that is mental retardation. Where I was thinking primarily custodially, I am now thinking more positively and creatively. (Third-year psychiatric resident.)

I learned about the different referral agencies and how they operate but many aspects did not apply to me since I only work with mildly mentally retarded. (Vocational rehabilitation counselor with a caseload of mentally retarded clients in the community.)

This experience has helped me to realize how limited our knowledge is in the area of mental retardation, that the field is wide open for experimentation and new approaches—I came looking for answers, and for me to accept that there are certain guidelines only was quite reassuring. This provides the stimuli to seek my own level of functioning with the retarded. (Psychiatric social worker in mental retardation service of community mental health program.)

I expect to be changing jobs in the near future and will be working with the mentally retarded. (Psychiatric social worker serving patients on leave from state hospitals for the mentally ill.)

I feel it is encouraging to hear other professionals express similar concerns which reassures me that some of my frustration and impatience is a product of the *field* in addition to my problems and my agency's shortcomings. (Chief social worker, private mental retardation hospital.)

I have gained some hope and enthusiasm that I did not have when I started the course. It's the old bureaucratic rut that kills imagination and burns up enthusiasm and I was in it quite deeply. You get an idea of what needs to be done but you turn to go about meeting the needs and the obstacles appear insurmountable. I will keep trying to see to it that these needs are met though. (Psychiatric social worker serving mentally ill and mentally retarded patients on leave from state hospitals.)

Increased my hope for eventual improvement of the mentally retarded under proper treatment methods. (Physician in charge of ward in a state mental retardation hospital.)

I will be more relaxed in my work with the retarded—I have been reassured that what I am doing is not detrimental to their well-being. (Social workers in Regional Diagnostic and Counseling Center for the Mentally Retarded.)

I now know there is not only work to be done in the community, but also in our professional status. I am amazed at the lack of true emotional feeling about people, our retarded. How can true authorities in this field be truly knowledgeable if they have lost contact with the people involved? (Nurse, administrator of private mental retardation hospital.)

Even though I learned different ways in which I could be instrumental in improvement of programming I also had some very strong negative feelings in the manner in which the mentally retarded are treated. . . . This experience has assisted me to recognize where I will be of most value—that is out in the community organizing parents to take part in the determination of their own mental health needs—*primary prevention* being the most important to me. (Social worker in Regional Diagnostic and Counseling Center for the Mentally Retarded.)

Following are some responses to another question, "What suggestions do you have for improving the course in the future?"

If the content is continually adjusted for current problems and emerging changes, I see little other need for improvement. (School teacher in state mental retardation hospital.)

We need more variety in the make-up of those attending, i.e. nursing care and paraprofessional people without degrees. (Social worker in state mental retardation hospital.)

More active student participation. (Clinical psychologist in mental retardation service of a community mental health program.)

I would like to hear more of the research that is going on in this field and have wished that we could come to grips with the Lanterman Mental Retardation Act of 1969 (California), current political philosophy relating to our field, and much more to do with the legislators themselves as they view mental retardation. . . . (Psychiatric social worker with caseload of patients on leave from state hospitals for the mentally retarded.)

More consistency and elaboration of particular topics. For example: the role of the county in psychiatric treatment of the mentally retarded could be explored with regard to its relation to other services in the county or in the State. (Clinical psychologist in a state hospital for the mentally ill.)

Reactions of the Mental Retardation Course Coordinator

In addition to the above responses as to the effect of the training, the following are the author's personal reactions to the impact of the courses on the trainees.

1. A substantial number of professionals have received training in the delivery of mental health services to the mentally retarded. Every effort has been made to keep the training practical and related to the immediate working problems of the trainee.

2. These professionals have developed a greater appreciation of the multifactorial nature of mental retardation, and of the functions of psychiatric and nonpsychiatric agencies and personnel in providing mental health services to the retarded.

3. Through active participation in field work experiences under supervision, and through regular discussions with preceptors, trainees have been enabled to more effectively deliver mental health services to the mentally retarded in their own agencies, and they have been able to share their learning with their colleagues, thereby greatly expanding the impact of the Center's training program in mental retardation.

A PROGRESS NOTE

During the Spring 1971 quarter, the writer initiated a series of discussion sessions involving representatives of various public and private agencies providing mental health services to the mentally retarded for the purpose of a) defining training needs of professionals in the field, and b) indicating ways in which the Center could meet these needs. It was generally agreed that the existing mental retardation courses at the Center were meeting some needs of professional practitioners in mental retardation although, as pointed out in the section on trainee's comments, many changes could be considered to make the training more useful and relevant.

The discussions also indicated that there were at least three other groups whose training needs were not being met. One was management-level administrators of mental retardation programs, whether in institutional or community settings. A second group were the paraprofessionals such as family caretakers, volunteers, aides. A third was "enlightened citizens" such as members of boards for planning and implementing mental retardation programs and services, legislators, and other influential persons on whose support the success of a program often rests.

Accordingly, at the time of present writing, several task forces have been working to develop goals, objectives, methods, and evaluation approaches to meet the training needs of these various "consumer" groups. Each task force is developing proposals which may lead to expanded training opportunities. A key feature of this process is the active participation of the "consumers," who will be using the training, in the planning and development of the training itself. The writer is firmly convinced that this process of dynamic involvement will eventually contribute much to raising the level of competency in the delivery of mental health services to the mentally retarded.

REFERENCES

1. Hume, Portia Bell: General principles of community psychiatry. In Arieti, S. (Ed.): *American Handbook of Psychiatry.* New York, Basic Books, Inc., 1966. Vol. III, pp. 515-541.
2. Katz, Elias: *The Retarded Adult in the Community.* Springfield, Illinois, Thomas, 1968, Chap. X and XI.

Appendix

SCHEDULE OF SEMINARS FOR THE MENTAL RETARDATION COURSES*

CENTER FOR TRAINING IN COMMUNITY PSYCHIATRY
AND MENTAL HEALTH ADMINISTRATION AT BERKELEY
2045 Dwight Way, Berkeley, California 94704

Community Psychiatry 101-E
Introduction to Mental Health Services for the Mentally Retarded

Time: Monday, Tuesday, Wednesday, Thursday, and Friday, 9:30 AM
to 5:30 PM

7/13/70 (10:30 AM-12M)	1. Introduction to the Four Courses in the Mental Retardation Sequence—Portia Bell Hume, M.D., Elias Katz, Ph.D.
7/13/70 (3:00-5:30 PM)	2. Direct and Indirect Services on Behalf of the Mentally Retarded in a Comprehensive Mental Health Program—Portia Bell Hume, M.D.
7/14/70 (9:30 AM-12M)	3. Definitions; Classifications; Epidemiology of Mental Retardation; History of Services for the Mentally Retarded—Elias Katz, Ph.D.
7/14/70 (3:00-5:30 PM)	4. Mental Health Services for the Mentally Retarded (I): State Level—William C. Keating, Jr., M.D.
7/15/70 (9:30 AM-12M)	5. Field Trip—Children's Health Home, San Mateo
7/15/70 (1:30-4:00 PM)	6. Field Trip—Agnews State Hospital
7/16/70 (9:30 AM-12M)	7. Mental Health Services for the Mentally Retarded (II): County Level—Ernest F. Pecci, M.D.; Leonti H. Thompson, M.D.
7/16/70	8. Mental Health Services for the Mentally Re-

---

* Courses offered during Summer, 1970; Fall, 1970; Winter, 1971; and Spring,
1971.

(3:00-5:30 PM)	tarded (III): Regional Centers—Charles A. Gardipee, M.D.; Edgar F. Pye, M.S.W.
7/17/70 (9:30 AM-12M)	9. Relationship of Biological and Genetic Factors to the Mental Health of the Mentally Retarded —Peter Cohen, M.D.
7/17/70 (3:00-5:30 PM)	10. Relationship of Socioeconomic Factors to the Mental Health of the Mentally Retarded with Special Reference to Poverty and Mental Retardation—Harold E. Dent, Ph.D.
7/20/70 (9:30 AM-12M)	11. Field Trip—Multipurpose Center, Contra Costa County
7/20/70 (1:30-4:00 PM)	12. Field Trip—Walnut Creek Work Training Center
7/21/70 (9:30 AM-12M)	13. Field Trip—San Francisco Recreation Center for Handicapped
7/21/70 (1:30-4:00 PM)	14. Field Trip—SFARC Social Development Program
7/22/70 (9:30 AM-12M)	15. Problems in Differential Diagnosis and Evaluation of Mental Retardation and Mental Illness— George F. Hexter, M.D.
7/22/70 (3:00-5:30 PM)	16. Treatment of Behavioral Disturbances in the Severely Mentally Retarded—Nathan Miron, Ph.D.
(9:30-11:30 AM) 7/23/70	17. Field Trip—Alameda County Mental Retardation Service
7/23/70 (12:30 PM)	Luncheon at EBARC Work-Training Center, Berkeley
(1:30-4:00 PM)	18. Field Trip—EBARC Work-Training Center, Berkeley
7/24/70 (9:30 AM-12M)	19. Counseling and Psychotherapy with the Mentally Retarded and Their Families (I)—Charlyne Nowik, M.D.
7/24/70 (3:00-5:30 PM)	20. Counseling and Psychotherapy with the Mentally Retarded and Their Families (II)—Charles M. Moody, M.S.W.

Workshops: 1:00 to 2:45 PM in groups each with a preceptor.

Purpose: To prepare trainee for field work placement.

7/13/70	1. Trainee discusses areas of interest with preceptor as a basis for selecting appropriate field work required by subsequent courses in this sequence.

| 7/14/70 | 2. Trainee develops purposes of field work project. Role of trainee's field work. |

7/14/70   2. Trainee develops purposes of field work project. Role of trainee's field work.

7/16/70   3. Discussion of plans for field work project. Role of trainee's field work supervisor. Role of Center preceptor.

7/17/70   4. Discussion of plans for field work project.

7/21/70   5. Evaluation of field work project.

7/24/70   6. Discussion of field work project.

* * *

Community Psychiatry 102-E
Methods of Delivering Mental Health Services to the
Mentally Retarded

Schedule of Seminars (4 to 6 PM)

9/28/70   1. Professional Roles in Working with Parents of the Retarded—James M. Eason, M.S.W.; Marion Hanlon, M.D.; Edgar F. Pye, M.S.W.

10/5/70   2. Team Approach in a Developmental Evaluation Unit —Doris Bradley, M.S.W.

10/19/70   3. Psychotherapy with the Mentally Retarded and Their Families—Ernest F. Pecci, M.D.

10/26/70   4. Mental Health Services for Emotionally Disturbed, Retarded Children and Their Parents in a Preschool Program—Helen Huggins

11/2/70   5. Counseling Services to Emotionally Disturbed, Retarded Students in a Public School Guidance Program—Alice Henry, M.A.

11/9/70   6. Progress Reports on Field Work by Trainees

11/16/70   7. Mental Health Functions of Recreation and Physical Fitness for the Mentally Retarded—Janet Pomeroy, M.S.

11/23/70   8. Indirect Services: Mental Health Consultation to Agencies Serving the Mentally Retarded—R. K. Janmeja Singh, Ph.D.

11/30/70   9. Pastoral Counseling of the Mentally Retarded and Their Families—Chaplain Moffett Dennis

12/7/70   10. Mental Health Functions of Rehabilitation Counselors with Retarded Clients—Louis Kamen, M.A.

12/4/70   11. Progress Reports on Field Work by Trainees

* * *

Community Psychiatry 103-E
Agency Approaches to the Delivery of Mental Health Services to the Mentally Retarded

Schedule of Seminars (4 to 6 PM)

1/4/71	1. Contra Costa County Mental Health Services: Multipurpose Centers for the Mentally Retarded—Ernest F. Pecci, M.D.
1/11/71	2. San Francisco City and County Mental Health Services: Mental Retardation Team—Marjorie S. Baker, Ph.D., Carolyn M. Goldrath, M.S.W.; John M. Williams, M.D.
1/18/71	3. Alameda County Mental Health Services: Mental Retardation Services—Virginia Blacklidge, M.D.
1/25/71	4. Golden Gate Regional Diagnostic and Counseling Center for the Mentally Retarded—Peter Cohen, M.D.; Edgar F. Pye, M.S.W.
2/1/71	5. Progress Reports on Field Work by Trainees
2/8/71	6. Sonoma State hospital—George Butler, M.D.
2/15/71	Holiday
2/22/71	7. Agnews State Hospital's Mental Retardation Program: A Joint Program of the State Departments of Mental Hygiene and Rehabilitation—Harold W. Nolen, Jr., M.D.; Ted Cutting, B.A.
3/1/71	8. Cooperative Programs of the Department of Rehabilitation and the Department of Education for School Work-Programs with Mentally Retarded Students—L. Wayne Campbell, M.A.; Dennis Dunne, M.A.
3/8/71	9. Mental Health Services for Mentally Retarded Students in an Urban Public School Setting—Robert W. Whitenack, Jr., M.A.
3/15/71 (2:30-4 PM)	10. Progress Reports on Field Work by Trainees
3/15/71 (4-6 PM)	11. Mental Health Services for the Mentally Retarded Through Sheltered Workshops and Activity Centers —Douglas Anderson, M.S.W.
3/22/71 (2:30-4 PM)	12. Progress Reports on Field Work by Trainees
3/22/71 (4-6 PM)	13. How a Lekotek Was Started and How It Works— Karin Stensland Junker, Ph.D.

✳   ✳   ✳

Community Psychiatry 104-E
Recent Developments in Hental Health Services for the
Mentally Retarded

Schedule of Seminars (4 to 6 PM)

4/5/71	1. Mental Health of the Mentally Retarded at Fairview State Hospital—Irving Stone, M.A.
4/12/71	2. Behavior Modification: Techniques with the Mentally Retarded—David Loberg, Ph.D.; Nathan Miron, Ph.D.
4/19/71	3. Development Centers for Handicapped Minors and Foster Grandparents: Their Impact on the Mental Health of the Mentally Retarded—Henry A. Caruso, M.A.
4/26/71	4. Training Programs for Family Caretakers of the Mentally Retarded—Richard A. Mamula, M.S.W.
5/3/71	5. Creative Art Expression as Therapy for the Mentally Retarded—Florence Ludins-Katz, M.A.
5/10/71	6. Progress Reports on Field Work by Trainees
5/17/71	7. The "Six-hour" Retarded Child—Ralph C. Kennedy, M.D.
5/24/71	8. Sex Education and Planned Parenthood—Paul Gardner, M.S.W.; John C. McIvor, B.A.; Charles C. Moody, M.S.W.
6/7/71	9. Statewide Delivery of Services to the Mentally Retarded—Dennis G. Amundson, B.S. and Staff
6/14/71	10. New Perspectives in the Delivery of Mental Health Services to the Mentally Retarded—Elias Katz, Ph.D.
6/21/71	11. Progress Reports on Field Work by Trainees

NAME INDEX

265

SUBJECT INDEX